ISBN: 978-0-9556746-2-4

Published by Apply2 Ltd
Chelsea House, Chelsea Street, New Basford,
Nottingham, NG7 7HN.

Prepared by:
York Publishing Services Ltd
64 Hallfield Road
Layerthorpe
York
YO31 7ZQ
Tel: 01904 431213 Website: www.yps-publishing.co.uk

Testimonials from Previous Prospective Medical Students

'I found the guide really helpful and actually being able to practice the questions with the mock test really helped improved my confidence'

LS, Fife

'Thanks for all your help – the guide was excellent and would recommend it to anyone'

ND, Norwich

'I was really panicking about my UKCAT but your guide helped me prepare so that when I did the exam I was relaxed and knew what to expect – thankyou!'

PM, London

'Brilliant – No – Excellent guide. Would highly recommend it to anyone who wants to do well in their UKCAT'

CP, Nottingham

'Sat the UKCAT last week and I have to say that if I had not worked through your guide I would not have done nearly as well – will let you know my result when I get it'

MT, Cornwall

Other books in the Appy2 range available at www.apply2medicine.co.uk or www.apply2dentistry.co.uk:

'The Apply2Medicine Guide to Writing your Medical School Personal Statement: Your Way, Successfully'

This engaging, easy to use and comprehensive guide covers every aspect involved in the planning, writing and refining of your medical school Personal Statement. Aimed at school leavers, graduates and mature individuals applying to medical school, together with parents and teachers, this guide will help you to write a compelling and convincing medical school Personal Statement.

'Succeeding at Your Medical School Interview'

'Succeeding at Your Medical School Interview' sets out the principles for success. The book highlights the importance of preparation – 'Your Homework' – and provides a framework through which you can effectively handle any question from the interview panel.

'Becoming a Doctor: Is Medicine Really the Career for You?'

Is Medicine really the career for you? Do you really want to be a Doctor? If you want answers to these questions then read Apply2Medicine's no-nonsense guide to finding out more about becoming a Doctor and what a career in medicine really entails.

Contents

About the Authors

Matt Green, BSc (Hons), MPhil

After completing his BSc in Biochemistry Matt went on to complete an MPhil at the Royal Marsden Hospital in London. This involved working closely with medical professionals on a number of projects developing novel drugs for the treatment of ovarian cancer. After setting up a private tuition service in 2004, Matt went on to found Apply2Medicine in 2005, and has been working to help prospective medical and dental students secure their first choice University place for the last four years.

Jemini Jethwa, BSc (Hons), MSc

After completing a BSc in Human Psychology, Jemini went on to complete an MSc in Occupational Psychology at the University of Nottingham. Following extensive experience of compiling psychometric and aptitude tests over the course of her Masters degree, Jemini has been helping prospective medical and dentistry school students revise for the UKCAT since April 2007.

Acknowledgements

We would like to thank all those who provided such valuable feedback in relation to our UKCAT revision exercises.

Preface

The aim of this guide is to help you to prepare yourself fully for your approaching UKCAT. With the introduction of this test for the majority of UK Medical and Dental Schools, applicants need to ensure that they are more prepared than ever to succeed in their application.

This guide addresses each of the five sections of the UKCAT, providing the reasoning behind each section of the test, together with example questions.

This guide culminates in an entire mock UKCAT test that you should complete under timed conditions. To gain the full benefit of this guide we recommend that you visit our website to download a free answer sheet to use when working through the example and mock test questions in this guide (www.apply2medicine.co.uk/ukcat or www.apply2dentistry.co.uk/ukcat). If you feel that you still require further practice after working through the examples and mock test contained within this guide, you can visit the above websites to subscribe to further online tests.

From all at Apply2.co.uk we would like to wish you the best of luck with your application to Medical or Dental School.

Chapter 1

Introduction to the UKCAT

What is the UKCAT?

The UK Clinical Aptitude Test (UKCAT) is an aptitude test used as part of the selection process by a group of UK university Medical and Dental schools. The test has been devised in order to help universities further distinguish from the many applicants who apply for Medical or Dental programmes.

Candidates who apply to study Medicine or Dentistry will not only have to have excelled academically, they will also need to posses the relevant mental abilities, attitudes, views, perceptions and professional behaviours which are required to be effective Doctors or Dentists.

The UKCAT provides universities with better information to enable them to select candidates of the highest calibre to progress successfully within the field of Medicine or Dentistry. The UKCAT enables the elimination of unsuitable candidates at an early stage in the selection process, by testing for a number of skills and competencies, for example a candidate's ability to make decisions based on limited information.

The UKCAT, which is computer rather than paper based, is co-ordinated by the UKCAT consortium important to note that the UKCAT does not have a pass rate. Your UKCAT results are used together with other factors such as your Personal Statement and predicted grades as an overall indicator of your suitability for a career in Medicine or Dentistry. Each University sets it own parameters as to how and to what degree the UKCAT results are used as part of the selection process. For example, some Universities rank candidates based on the subtest with the lowest score whereas others base their decision on the average score of the candidate.

Eligibility for the UKCAT

The UKCAT was formally adopted in 2006 and is now used by twenty-six Medical and Dental schools in the UK (listed below). The requirement for applicants to complete the UKCAT applies to all UK, EU and the majority of international applicants. Test centers exist worldwide, including in most EU countries. Registration for the test is made online at www.ukcat.ac.uk.

Registering for the UKCAT

Registration for the 2008 UKCAT starts at the beginning of May 2008 via an online process. We would strongly recommend that you strive to sit the UKCAT at a time that does not impact on your studies if applicable, ideally during the summer. There is also an incentive of the test fee being reduced if you complete the test before the end of August 2008. If you do not take the UKCAT test before the deadline, your application will be automatically rejected, and you will have to reapply the following year.

Candidates who are intending to apply in 2008 for entry to the following Universities in 2009 or for deferred entry in 2010 are required to complete the UKCAT before the middle of October 2008 (exact date can be confirmed on the UKCAT website). The results from your test are only valid in the year the test is taken. If your application to Medicine or Dentistry is not successful and you re-apply the following year you will have to re-sit the UKCAT.

If you have any special circumstances, such as a disability or illness, you may be provided with extra time to complete the test. However, you will need to give details of such circumstances at the time of registration, and provide evidence to substantiate this. There are two versions of the UKCAT, the Standard and the Special Education Needs (SEN) version, which is the same test with extra time allowed for completion.

List of participating Universities for the UKCAT

University of Aberdeen
Brighton and Sussex Medical School
Cardiff University
University of Dundee
University of Durham
University of East Anglia
University of Edinburgh
University of Glasgow
Hull York Medical School
Keele University
King's College London
Imperial College London Graduate Entry

University of Leeds
University of Leicester
University of Manchester
University of Newcastle
University of Nottingham
University of Oxford Graduate Entry
Peninsula Medical School
Queen Mary, University of London
Queen's University Belfast
University of Sheffield
University of Southampton
University of St Andrews
St George's, University of London
Warwick University Graduate Entry

How do I prepare?

Although it is stated that you cannot prepare for the UKCAT, this is simply not the case. Through completing practice tests you will have a clearer idea of what to expect and feel more confident. We would encourage you to read carefully through the UKCAT website so that you have a clear understanding of the test process and the interface that is used in the test centre.

To ensure that you are fully prepared for your UKCAT, work through this book and practice what you have learnt by completing the mock test (see Chapter 8) under timed conditions. The first part of this guide explains each sub-test of the UKCAT, why it used and provides practice questions for you to work through to ensure that you put into practice what you have learnt.

The second part of this guide comprises a full mock test that you can work through under timed conditions.

We would recommend that you visit our website to download our free answer sheet, which will make it easier to refer your answers back to the guide. There are also further mock tests available on our websites.

Chapter 2

Succeeding in the UKCAT

Practice makes perfect

As with any test it is essential to practice example questions to ensure you are familiar with the structure and type of content you will be tested on. The UKCAT is no exception despite what people may tell you!

The following chapters will enable you to practice each of the different subsections which together form the UKCAT. Each chapter contains questions equivalent to half of what you would be faced with in the test, designed to help you to put into practice what you learn. This will enable you to familiarise yourself with the format and style of the UKCAT and hopefully help you to realise that most of the questions in the test will be of general ability.

However, this is not to say that the UKCAT test is of an easy nature, otherwise it would not be a useful tool in the selection process. Although the UKCAT may measure general ability you will find that you only have a limited amount of time for each subsection.

Each of the subtests are individually timed, therefore it is not possible for you to make up for lost time in the other remaining subtests. It is vital that you complete each section fully as you progress through the test and do not leave any questions unanswered. By doing so, if you find that you do not have time to go back and check your answers, you will at least stand a chance of scoring a mark.

It may therefore be more valuable to time yourself when you undertake the mock test at the end of this book. This way you will be able to enhance your time management skills, together with increasing your confidence and also alleviate any anxiety you may have. The aim of this book is to ensure that, on the day of your test, you are faced with something you are already familiar with.

This book culminates with a full mock test for you to complete under timed conditions. An answer sheet can be downloaded for free from www.apply2.co.uk to help you make the most of this book.

What are multiple choice tests?

The UKCAT is set out in a multiple choice format. Multiple choice tests are commonly used within the field of selection and assessment. The test questions are designed to test a candidate's awareness and understanding of a particular subject.

The subtests within the UKCAT are based on an answer format known as *'A-Type Questions'*, which is the most commonly used design in multiple choice tests. This specific design helps to make transparent the number of choices which need to be selected. These questions usually consist of a *'Stem and lead-in question'* which are followed by a *'series'* of *'choices'*. To illustrate this, below is an example of a Quantitative Reasoning question:

Stem

This is generally an introductory statement, question or passage of relevant information which elicits the correct answer. The stem on the whole provides all the information for the question or questions which will follow e.g.

'There are 100 students who go on a school trip to a science park.'

Lead-in Question

This is the question which identifies the exact answer e.g.

'35% of the students were female, how many female students were there?'

Choices

In a multiple choice test, the choices will generally consist of one correct answer. However, depending on the type of question, you may be required to select two or even three correct answers. Wherever there are correct answers there are also incorrect answers, which are also known as the *'distracters'*. For the above example, typical choices could be as follows:

A. 25

B. 67

C. **35 – Correct answer (35% of 100 students = 35 female students)**

D. 65

General tips for answering multiple choice tests

- Read, and **re-read the question** to ensure you fully understand what is being asked, not what you want to be asked.

- **Eliminate any incorrect answers** you know are wrong.

- Read the question and try to answer it before looking at the choices available to you.

- **Do not spend too much time on one question** – remember you only have a set amount of time per section so, as a rule of thumb, you should spend x amount per question (x = time of section ÷ number of questions).

- **Do not keep changing your mind** – research has shown that the first answer that appeals to you is often the correct one.

- If you cannot decide between two answers, look carefully and decide whether for one of the options you are making an unnecessary assumption – **trust your gut instinct.**

- Always select an answer for a given question even if you do not know the answer – **never leave any answers blank.**

- **Pace yourself** – you will need to work through the test at the right speed. Too fast and your accuracy may suffer, too slow and you may run out of time. Use this guide to practice your time keeping and approach to answering each question – you need to do what works for you, not what might work for someone else.

- In the actual test, you will be given the opportunity to mark your questions for review, so do try to remember and **go back and check** that you have answered all the questions to the best of your ability.

- To familiarise yourself with the way the online test will be conducted visit the **online testing demonstration** which is available on the UKCAT website.

- Remember you will only be awarded marks for correct answers, and marks will not be deducted for incorrect answers. Therefore try to **answer every single question**, even ones you are unsure of.

- When you take the test, listen carefully to the administrator's instructions.

- If you are unsure about anything, remember to ask the test administrator before the test begins. Once the clock begins ticking, interruptions will not be allowed.

- You may be presented with a question which you simply cannot answer due to difficulty or if the wording is too vague. If you have only twenty seconds per question, and you find yourself spending five minutes determining the answer for each question then your time management skills are poor and you are wasting valuable time.

Chapter 3

The Verbal Reasoning Subtest

The purpose of the UKCAT Verbal Reasoning subtest is to assess a candidate's ability to read and critically evaluate passages of written information which cover a variety of topics, including both scientific and non-scientific themes. The Verbal Reasoning subtest used in the UKCAT is a classic critical thinking and reasoning test. Critical reasoning and critical thinking are core skills which are required to achieve understanding of complex arguments, evaluate different perceptions and find solutions to problems.

Achieving high scores in the Verbal Reasoning subtest reflects a candidate's ability to interpret written information within the workplace based on the facts you are presented with, rather than letting your personal knowledge influence your decision, an essential skill required when working within a healthcare setting.

The following qualities are required to enable effective critical thinking and critical reasoning:

- The ability to differentiate between fact and opinion.

- The ability to examine and differentiate between assumptions, both those presented in the text and your own.

- The ability to be open minded but also flexible as you explore explanations, causes and solutions to various problems – without your own bias.

- Awareness of misleading arguments, which consist of vague and manipulative reasoning.

- The ability to remain focused on the overall picture while investigating specifics based on the information present.

- The ability to discover reputable sources.

The Verbal Reasoning subtest in the UKCAT consists of eleven stems or passages of written information. Each passage comprises of four lead-in questions/statements, which in total equal forty-four items to complete. For each answer you will have three options: 'True', 'False' or 'Can't tell'. You will be allocated twenty-two minutes to complete this section, which includes one minute administration time, which equates to thirty seconds per question.

For each of the stems, you will be faced with a passage which has been extracted from various sources. These passages do not contain any curriculum content. However, the purpose of each of the passages is to try and persuade the reader to adopt a specific view of an argument. **<u>The key to approaching Verbal Reasoning questions is to base your decision purely on the information and facts provided in the passages</u>**. You must avoid using any previous knowledge you may have regarding each subject to bias your answer. The aim of the Verbal Reasoning subtest is to read the passage, and evaluate the four corresponding statements, according to the following rules:

True – if you consider the statement to be true based on the information provided in the passage.

False – if you consider the statement to be false based on the information provided in the passage.

Can't tell – if you cannot state whether the statement is true or false without further information which is not provided.

Summary of Verbal Reasoning structure

Stem

The stem will consist of a series of passages, extracted from various different sources such as leaflets, magazines, newspaper articles, and various other sources of written information. The Verbal Reasoning subtest consists of eleven stems.

Lead-in question

Each of the stems will consist of four separate lead-in questions which are related to the stem in some way. Therefore there will be a total of forty-four lead-in questions.

Choices

Your task will be to decide whether the lead-in question is 'True', 'False' or 'Can't tell' based purely on the evidence given in the passages or stems.

Time limit = twenty-two minutes. Therefore you will have thirty seconds per question.

When you are working through the UKCAT subtests it can be counter-productive to monitor exactly how long you spend on answering each question, especially when you need to read through and digest the information presented in the stem. Therefore a more useful time management approach is to divide each subtest into four quarters. So, in the case of the Verbal Reasoning subtest, after approximately six minutes you should be working on the fourth passage, after approximately eleven minutes you should be commencing the seventh passage and so on. If you find yourself falling behind at these points you know that you need to pick up the pace.

Example of a Verbal Reasoning question

> *It has been a controversial debate that half of the jobs which Labour created in 1997 have been filled by foreign workers. The Department of Work and Pensions claims that over 52% of jobs have gone to foreign workers. One recent 'eye-opener' has been that the government have declared that more than 1.1 million overseas workers have come to Britain in the past 10 years, and not 8 million as previously disclosed.*
>
> *National statistics provided by the Home Office indicate that 1.5 million overseas workers have entered the UK over the last decade. However, in reply to this the Department of Work and Pensions has claimed that the extra 400,000 workers were British residents who were born overseas. With such statistics the findings seem to make a mockery of what the government had initially proposed – 'British jobs for every British worker'.*

A   48% of jobs have gone to British workers.

Answer: True, False or Can't tell

Verbal Reasoning hints and tips

- **<u>Ensure the answer you give is determined solely by the information contained within the passage and not your assumptions.</u>**

- Look out for misleading words such as *'all'*, *'everything'* and *'completely'* – these are specific types of words which suggest that the whole of a particular object, person, area or group are wholly affected.

- Other misleading words include *'virtually'*, 'almost', *'particularly'*, *'nearly'* and *'close to'* – these are words which refer to something *close to* happening rather than actually happening.

- It is very important that you **<u>read the passages very carefully</u>**. One common mistake that candidates often make is to allow their previous knowledge on a subject to interfere with and bias the information and facts that are presented in the passages (often these are of a conflicting nature).

- Remember that each of the passages are **<u>deliberately manipulated to influence the candidate</u>** to a particular perspective or point of view.

- Often you may find that a passage states information which may subsequently alter or be contradicted further on in the passage. Ensure that you note any changes or contradictions and reflect these when selecting your answers.

- **<u>Do not waste too much time thinking about a difficult question</u>**. All questions are marked equally, therefore a difficult question will not be worth more than an easy question and vice versa. If you having difficulty understanding a passage, flag it and move on to the next passage, ensuring to come back to it later.

- Remember **<u>time management is key throughout</u>** the test and in the Verbal Reasoning subtest you should spend no longer than thirty seconds considering an answer.

- If you find a question particularly difficult you can flag it so that you can return to it before you move onto the next subtest – when flagging a question to return to we recommend that you still select an answer in case you do not have time to return to the question.

- **<u>Attempt all questions</u>** as you will not be penalised for getting questions wrong, but you will lose marks if you leave an answer blank.

- Learn to **<u>manage your time efficiently</u>**. Go through practise mock papers and time yourself as if you were in a real exam. By familiarising yourself with the types of questions you will be faced with you will be able to analyse where your weaknesses are and improve.

- Read through newspapers and various other sources of literature which use elaborate and detailed language. This will enhance your skills in reading and also enable you to consider in-depth critical arguments and perspectives.

7 simple steps to Verbal Reasoning

Step 1

Browse through the passages (answering each question systematically) and try to gain a feel for what the passage is trying to portray. Remember not to let previous knowledge on a subject interfere with what is actually presented in the passage.

Step 2

Note down any changes or contradictions in terms of information or valid points.

Step 3

Read through each question and determine exactly what you are being asked.

Step 4

Read through the passage again if necessary and answer each of the questions. Remember to take into account previous notes.

Step 5

Eliminate answers which are obviously incorrect.

Step 6

Try to answer the questions as accurately as possible and do not leave any answers blank, even if you are not sure of the answer.

Step 7

If you are having trouble answering any of the questions still select an answer and flag it so you can return to it later.

Verbal Reasoning practice examples

The following part of this chapter will enable you to work through various examples of Verbal Reasoning questions together with evaluating your answers against explanations. Remember, you can download a free answer sheet from www.apply2.co.uk to make it easier for you when working through these examples.

Example 1

> *A virus-laden cream, to prevent the spread of MRSA, could be made available within the next two years. Scientists are at a highly advanced stage of developing the cream, which contains a combination of various viruses which target the MRSA bug. The cream is to be applied inside the noses of hospital patients. Once in the nose the viruses will fasten themselves onto the MRSA bacteria, and infuse the MRSA bacteria with their own genetic material. It has been proposed that viruses reproduce themselves, which suggests that repeated treatments may not be necessary, when compared to other treatments. The virus cream seems to be one of the latest ongoing examples of a resurgence of interest in bacteriophage viruses. It has been proposed that this specific form of treatment, involving the use of bacteriophages, may be a potential solution to the increasing problem of bacterial resistance to antibiotics.*

1   There is fragmentary curiosity in the treatment of viruses through methods involving the use of bacteria

2 MRSA is a deadly viral disease

3 Viruses tend to replicate themselves, which may mean that treatments will be incessant

4 Bacterial treatment is a possible, but not yet realised solution to the mounting problem of virus resistance to antibiotics

Example 2

> *The internet is a convenient place to search for vast amounts of information and to conduct online shopping. However, it has been noted that there is an increased rate of fraud when individuals have purchased items over the internet. The two most popular types of fraud perpetrated on the internet are 'Rogue Trading' and 'Identity Fraud'. Rogue trading is attempted by dishonest individuals who may advertise their items using false descriptions. There may actually be cases where the items do not even exist. Rogue traders are also deceitful when they purposely advertise items without delivery or transportation rates. These rates are then revealed towards the end of the buying process, by which time the individual's payment details may have been received and it may possibly be too late to cancel the transaction. Identity fraud occurs when fraudulent traders gain access to your personal details, such as your credit card number. In most cases an item is usually delivered, hence the buyer will also have to give details of their address. These two personal details combined usually make it easier for a fraudster to withdraw money from their victim's bank account.*

5   The internet is always a prudent place to search for information and to shop for goods

6   Fraud is universally prevalent on the internet

7   Fraudsters advertising items under false pretences is an illustration of identity deception

8   Internet fraud can be divided into two categories: 'Rogue Trading' and 'Identity Fraud'

Example 3

Over the past 100 years, the earth has warmed by 1°F. The greenhouse effect has been part of the earth's workings from the beginning. The greenhouse effect helps sunlight to reach planet earth through gases such as carbon dioxide and methane. The gases also help prevent some of the heat from radiating back into space. If the greenhouse effect did not exist, the earth would not be warm enough for life to form. However, the Industrial Economy has released large amounts of carbon dioxide and, as a result, the earth is becoming warmer at an accelerating rate. As the earth gets warmer, sea levels are also gradually increasing. The Arctic and Antarctic are also getting warmer. In addition to this, heat waves are becoming more prevalent, and droughts and fires are much more noticeable than they were 100 years ago.

9   If it was not for the Industrial Economy, there would be no effects of global warming

10 Inconsistent climate change is a by-product of the greenhouse effect

11 The melting of glaciers has caused an increase in sea water levels

12 Droughts and fires are caused by the greenhouse effect being disturbed

Example 4

The population of the United Kingdom is ageing. It has increased from 55.9 million in 1971 to 60.2 million in 2005. That is almost an eight percent increase. However, this change is not spread out evenly across all age groups. In the last thirty or so years, the population aged 65 or over has increased from 13 percent to 16 percent. Within this age group the proportion of the population aged '65 and over' and '85 and over' increased from 7 percent in the 1970s to 12 percent in 2005. However, the percentage of the population living under the age of 16 has declined from 25 percent in 1971 to 19 percent in 2005. Over the last thirty years, the mean age of the UK population increased from 34.1 years in 1971 to 38.8 in 2005. This ageing is principally due to fertility, although in recent times there has been a decrease in mortality rates, with particular emphasis on older ages.

13 Over the last three decades there has been a decrease in the population aged 65 and over

14 There has been a population increase of 4.3 million from the 1970s to 2005

15 Younger people are living much longer as they now have healthy lifestyles

16 There were more older people than younger people living in 2005

Example 5

> *The effects of smoking have been known for a very long time. The harmful and poisonous chemicals inside tobacco all have negative effects. If an individual smokes long-term they are more likely to suffer from the following: cancer, heart disease, blockage of vessels and so on. Since the 1st of July 2007, the UK government brought out new legislation which prohibited individuals from smoking in public places such as clubs, bars, pubs and restaurants. Many organisations have now incorporated a 'no smoking' policy within staff and customer areas. In order to advertise this policy, posters and pamphlets have been specifically put in staff canteens and customer waiting rooms. Many individuals have put forward their support, either by not smoking in these buildings, or by quitting smoking all together. However, a minority feel that this is an erosion of their freedom of choice.*

17 Due to the legislation enforced by the government many organisations now have a 'no smoking' policy

18 If an individual was to smoke for at least 10 years, they are more likely to suffer from cancer, heart disease, blockage of vessels and so on

19 All individuals seem to be supporting the 'no smoking' policy

20 Due to the enforcement of the 'no smoking' legislation, it will be up to the organisations to comply by the rules

Justifications of Verbal Reasoning practice examples

Example 1

> A virus-laden cream, to prevent the spread of MRSA, could be made available within the next two years. Scientists are at a highly advanced stage of developing the cream, which contains a combination of various viruses which target the MRSA bug. The cream is to be applied inside the noses of hospital patients. Once in the nose the viruses will fasten themselves onto the MRSA bacteria, and infuse the MRSA bacteria with their own genetic material. It has been proposed that viruses reproduce themselves, which suggests that repeated treatments may not be necessary, when compared to other treatments. The virus cream seems to be one of the latest ongoing examples of a resurgence of interest in bacteriophage viruses. It has been proposed that this specific form of treatment, involving the use of bacteriophages, may be a potential solution to the increasing problem of bacterial resistance to antibiotics.

1 *There is fragmentary curiosity in the treatment of viruses though methods of using bacteria*

   Answer: True

This statement simply states that there is ongoing interest in the treatment of viruses using bacteriophages. Therefore it is safe to say that the assumption made in the above statement is 'True'.

2 *MRSA is a deadly viral disease*

Answer: Can't tell

This statement suggests that the 'MRSA virus is a deadly virus'. However, in the passage there is not enough information to reach such a conclusion. Even though the passage has information about the potential cure for MRSA, the passage does not provide information about how deadly it is. Although you may personally know how dangerous the MRSA virus is, it is not specifically stated in the passage – therefore you are unable to determine the answer without further information.

3 *Viruses tend to replicate themselves, which may mean that treatments will be incessant*

Answer: False

The passage states that viruses tend to reproduce themselves, which means that continual treatments will not be necessary. The above statement is therefore false, as it claims that treatments will need to be incessant or continual.

4 *Bacterial treatment is a possible, but not yet realised solution to the mounting problem of virus resistance to antibiotics*

Answer: True

Towards the final section of the passage, which relates to the ongoing interest in the resurgence of bacteriophages, it states that this specific form of treatment may be a *possible* solution to the increasing problem of bacterial resistance to antibiotics. This therefore means that bacterial treatment is a possible solution to the mounting problem of virus resistance to antibiotics.

Example 2

> The internet is a convenient place to search for vast amounts of information and to conduct online shopping. However, it has been noted that there is an increased rate of fraud when individuals have purchased items over the internet. The two most popular types of fraud perpetrated on the internet are 'Rogue Trading' and 'Identity Fraud'. Rogue trading is attempted by dishonest individuals who may advertise their items using false descriptions. There may actually be cases where the items do not even exist. Rogue traders are also deceitful when they purposely advertise items without delivery or transportation rates. These rates are then revealed towards the end of the buying process, by which time the individual's payment details may have been received and it may possibly be too late to cancel the transaction. Identity fraud occurs when fraudulent traders gain access to your personal details, such as your credit card number. In most cases an item is usually delivered, hence the buyer will also have to give details of their address. These two personal details combined usually make it easier for a fraudster to withdraw money from their victim's bank account.

5 *The internet is always a prudent place to search for information and to shop for goods*

   Answer: False

From the beginning of the passage, it is stated that the internet is a convenient place to search for information. However, when we carefully consider the consequences, the internet also has its drawback of being a popular place for fraud. Hence the above statement is false.

6 *Fraud is universally prevalent on the internet*

Answer: Can't tell

The passage states that fraud is usually on the increase when individuals purchase items over the internet. However, there is no mention of how much of the internet is affected. The above statement claims that fraud is universally prevalent over the internet, although there is limited information in the given passage. Therefore we are unable to arrive at such a conclusion.

7 *Fraudsters advertising items under false pretences is an illustration of identity deception*

Answer: False

The passage states that 'Identity Fraud' is a term used when fraudsters gain access to personal details, such as credit cards and addresses. On the other hand, 'Rogue Traders' are individuals who advertise items under bogus descriptions, or items which do not exist. This therefore means that the statement above is false.

8 *Internet fraud can be divided into two categories: 'Rogue Trading' and 'Identity Fraud'*

Answer: False

The first part of the passage suggests that fraud is on the increase and that there are two popular forms of fraud – 'Rogue Trading' and 'Identity Fraud'. However, the passage does not claim that these two groups of fraud are the only categories.

Example 3

> *Over the past 100 years, the earth has warmed by 1°F. The greenhouse effect has been part of the earth's workings from the beginning. The greenhouse effect helps sunlight to reach planet earth through gases such as carbon dioxide and methane. The gases also help prevent some of the heat from radiating back into space. If the greenhouse effect did not exist, the earth would not be warm enough for life to form. However, the Industrial Economy has released large amounts of carbon dioxide and, as a result, the earth is becoming warmer at an accelerating rate. As the earth gets warmer, sea levels are also gradually increasing. The Arctic and Antarctic are also getting warmer. In addition to this, heat waves are becoming more prevalent, and droughts and fires are much more noticeable than they were 100 years ago.*

9 *If it was not for the Industrial Economy, there would be no effects of global warming*

  Answer: Can't tell

Although the passage gives an example of the reasons for global warming, we are unable to conclude that the Industrial Economy is the 'only reason' why global warming exists. There may be other contributing factors which are not noted in the passage. For that reason, we are unable to conclude that the Industrial Economy is the only contributing factor to global warming.

10 *Inconsistent climate change is a by-product of the greenhouse effect*

Answer: True

Towards the end of the passage examples of the various effects of global warming are noted, such as sea levels gradually increasing, the Antarctic getting warmer and the increase in heat waves. These are all various examples of climate change or the results of the earth getting warmer.

11 *The melting of glaciers has caused an increase in sea water levels*

Answer: Can't tell

As mentioned in the final lines of the passage, one of the consequences of global warming has been an increase in sea levels. Although we may know from our own experience this is due to the fact that glaciers have melted, causing a rise in sea levels, there is no further information given on the exact processes involved in causing the sea levels to rise. This is a good example of a common mistake made by candidates who use their own knowledge to make their decision, rather than the information they are presented with.

12 *Droughts and fires are caused by the greenhouse effect being disturbed*

Answer: True

It is stated in the passage that the 'greenhouse effect' has had many negative consequences, such as drought and fire. Hence the statement is true based on the information provided in the passage.

Example 4

> *The population of the United Kingdom is ageing. It has increased from 55.9 million in 1971 to 60.2 million in 2005. That is almost an eight percent increase. However, this change is not spread out evenly across all age groups. In the last thirty or so years, the population aged 65 or over has increased from 13 percent to 16 percent. Within this age group the proportion of the population aged '65 and over' and '85 and over' increased from 7 percent in the 1970s to 12 percent in 2005. However, the percentage of the population living under the age of 16 has declined from 25 percent in 1971 to 19 percent in 2005. Over the last thirty years, the mean age of the UK population increased from 34.1 years in 1971 to 38.8 in 2005. This ageing is principally due to fertility, although in recent times there has been a decrease in mortality rates, with particular emphasis on older ages.*

13 *Over the last three decades there has been a decrease in the population aged 65 and over*

Answer: False

The second paragraph in the passage specifically states that the UK population aged 65 years and over has increased, rather than decreased as suggested by the statement above, therefore the answer is false.

14 *There has been a population increase of 4.3 million from the 1970s to 2005*

Answer: True

This requires a simple method of mental arithmetic and reading the passage carefully. Towards the beginning of the passage it is stated that the mean age of the UK population increased from 55.9 million to 60.2 million. This equals a difference of 4.3 million.

15 *Younger people are living much longer as they now have healthy lifestyles*

Answer: Can't tell

In the passage it is stated that 'the percentage of the population living under the age of 16 has declined' therefore at first we may think that the statement is false. However, although the passage states that the percentage of the population aged 16 and under has dropped since 1971, there is no specific information provided to make such a conclusion to the above question.

16 *There were more older people than younger people living in 2005*

Answer: False

If you look at the fourth line of the passage, it states that the population for those aged 65 and over has increased from 13% to 16%, from the 1970s to 2005. However, those living under the age of 16 years has decreased from 25% to 19% from the 1970s to 2005.

Example 5

> The effects of smoking have been known for a very long time. The harmful and poisonous chemicals inside tobacco all have negative effects. If an individual smokes long-term they are more likely to suffer from the following: cancer, heart disease, blockage of vessels and so on. Since the 1st of July 2007, the UK government brought out new legislation which prohibited individuals from smoking in public places such as clubs, bars, pubs and restaurants. Many organisations have now incorporated a 'no smoking' policy within staff and customer areas. In order to advertise this policy, posters and pamphlets have been specifically put in staff canteens and customer waiting rooms. Many individuals have put forward their support, either by not smoking in these buildings, or by quitting smoking all together. However, a minority feel that this is an erosion of their freedom of choice.

17 *Due to the legislation enforced by the government many organisations now have a 'no smoking' policy*

Answer: True

At the beginning of the passage, it is stated that 'many organisations' have now adopted a 'no smoking' policy. Hence it is fair to say that this statement is true.

18 *If an individual was to smoke for at least 10 years, they are more likely to suffer from cancer, heart disease, blockage of vessels and so on*

Answer: Can't Tell

In the passage it states that long-term smokers are more likely to suffer from various diseases, such as cancer, heart disease, blockage of vessels and so on. However there is no information given on the definition of what 'long-term' is, or how many years are regarded as long-term, hence there is insufficient information given to make such a conclusion.

19 *All individuals seem to be supporting the 'no smoking' policy*

Answer: False

It is stated in the passage that there is a minority group who are not in favour of the 'no smoking' policy. This therefore falsifies the above statement, as not everyone supports the policy.

20 *Due to the enforcement of the 'no smoking' legislation, it will be up to the organisations to comply by the rules*

Answer: Can't tell

There is limited information given to make a claim that it is the responsibility of the organisation to comply with the rules. Although you may have knowledge that there is government legislation to comply with the 'no smoking' policy, it is not actually stated in the passage, hence there is insufficient information to make such a conclusion.

Chapter 4

The Quantitative Reasoning Subtest

The Quantitative Reasoning subtest of the UKCAT will assess a candidate's ability to solve numerical problems, interpret data and also assess their basic maths skills relating to real life scenarios. The aim of this subtest is to objectively assess a candidate's ability to analyse, interpret, and manipulate complex numerical data.

Achieving high scores in the Quantitative Reasoning subtest reflects a candidate's ability to manipulate numerical information, which is an essential skill required by Doctors or Dentists in their everyday practice.

Before you attempt to answer any Quantitative Reasoning questions it is important that you refresh your basic knowledge of the following topics:

- Addition
- Subtraction
- Multiplication
- Division
- Percentages
- Ratio

- Mean, median and mode
- Fractions
- Decimal numbers

Also, you need to be able to interpret:

- Pie charts
- Line Graphs
- Bar graphs
- Tables

The Quantitative Reasoning subtest contains ten stems comprising of various tables, charts and graphs, with a total of forty questions relating to them (four items per stem). You will have twenty-two minutes to complete this section which includes one minute for administration. You will therefore have thirty-three seconds to complete each question.

This chapter will illustrate various examples of the types of numerical questions you will face when you sit your UKCAT.

Summary of Quantitative Reasoning structure

Stem

The stem will consist of various tables, charts and graphs. There will be a total of ten stems in the UKCAT.

Lead-in Question

For each of the stems, there will be four separate lead-in questions. In total there will be forty lead-in questions which relate to the various charts, graphs and tables.

Choices

You will be given five different answer options which will be in the format of A, B, C, D and E. Only one choice is the correct answer, and the remaining choices are known as '*distracters*'.

Time limit = twenty-two minutes. Therefore you will have thirty seconds per question.

When you are working through the UKCAT subtests it can be counter-productive to monitor exactly how long you spend on answering each question, especially when you need to read through and digest the information presented in the stem. Therefore a more useful time management approach is to divide each subtest into four quarters. So, in the case of the Quantitative Reasoning subtest, after approximately six minutes you should be working on the fifth stem, after approximately eleven minutes you should be commencing the tenth stem and so on. If you find yourself falling behind at these points you know that you need to pick up the pace.

Example of a Quantitative Reasoning question

Examine the table below

Currency	Rate of exchange = Pounds Sterling (£)
American – Dollar	$1.59 = £1.00
Indian – Rupee	0.0856 R = £1.00
French – Franc	1.45 F = £1.00
Cuban – Peso	1.8 CUP = £1.00
Bangladeshi – Taka	0.6 BGL = £1.00

How much is $150 worth in Pounds Sterling (£)?

A £94.33

B £49.36

C £94.34

D £49.37

E £94.30

Quantitative Reasoning hints and tips

Refresh your memory by working through your GCSE and A level maths books to ensure you are familiar with the following:

- ◇ Addition and subtraction
- ◇ Multiplication and division
- ◇ Fractions and percentages
- ◇ Converting fractions, decimals and percentages

⟡ Determining mode, mean and median averages

⟡ Algebra

⟡ Decimals

⟡ Distance, time and speed triangles

⟡ Calculating area and perimeters

⟡ Analysing charts, bar charts, pie charts, frequency tables etc

⟡ Square and cube numbers

- **<u>Work through the questions systematically.</u>** You may find that a question refers to your previous answer(s).

- **<u>Work out all your calculations on the whiteboard provided</u>,** if there are errors you may be able to determine from your rough workings at what point you made a mistake.

- Go through the practice mock papers and **<u>identify your strengths and weaknesses</u>** early so you can improve on your weaknesses. For example, you may be better at completing algebra equations rather than fractions. You can then address your weaknesses.

- When answering questions which involve humans, remember to calculate your final answer to the nearest whole number as people cannot be represented as a decimal or a fraction! This may be an important point to take note of when converting percentages to actual numbers.

- One major pitfall is to select an option which you think is nearest to the answer. Often you will find that the majority of the options are very close to each other and may differ in terms of decimal points or a single digit which is either added or removed. Therefore it is very important to evaluate the answer options very carefully.

- Always answer questions in the correct metric units. For example, a question may ask you to calculate something in centimetres but then give your final answer in metres. Therefore it is important to **read each item very closely**.

- Some algebra questions may require you to calculate the answer of 'X'. Often this will be X on its own or sometimes the answer may require you to find X^3 or X^2. Therefore it is always important to **look at how the questions require you to give your final answer.**

- Remember to **time yourself as you complete the mock tests**. This will improve your time management skills, ensuring you have adequate time to answer every question.

- Try not to spend too long on one question. All marks are awarded equally in this section. If you are unsure of the answer select the best possible answer, flag the question and return to it. By selecting an answer you at least stand a chance of scoring a mark, even if you run out of time and are unable to return to the flagged question.

- Do not waste too much time on questions you are unsure of – flag them and return to them later. Always provide an answer for each question as you will not be penalised for getting an answer wrong, even if you guess. A guess means that you have a

25% chance of getting the mark, so it is better to guess than to leave the question blank!

- If you really are unsure about a question eliminate the obvious wrong answers and then make a calculated guess.

4 simple steps to answering Quantitative Reasoning questions

Step 1

Read the question carefully.

Step 2

Calculate your rough workings step-by-step using the whiteboard provided.

Step 3

Eliminate answers which are obviously incorrect from the five options.

Step 4

Mark the most accurate answer. (Remember to give your answer in the metric values as requested by the question).

Quantitative Reasoning practice examples

Example 1

Washing Machine Brands	Wholesale Price for a Lot of 13 (£)	Recommended Retail Price (RRP) per Unit (£)
A	6789	732.13
B	7685	699.29
C	8786	875.85
D	8790	723.12
E	9009	932.45
F	5789	678.92
G	9843	923.40

1   A store buys 11 'Brand G' washing machines at the relative wholesale price and sells them all at the recommended retail price. How much profit did the store make?

A   £1838.29

B   £1828.90

C   £1768.90

D   £1828.75

E   £1829.60

2   A store sold 7 'Brand D' washing machines with 25% off the recommended retail price. What loss did the store make?

   A £938.98

   B £1000.98

   →C £3796.38

   D £936.67

   E £937.60

3   By how much does the recommended retail price for 'Brand B' differ when compared to the wholesale price? Please give your answer as a percentage.

   A 16%

   B 18.3%

   C 25.3%

   D 15.3%

   E 15.9%

4   If a 'Brand C' washing machine was sold at 5/8th of the recommended retail price, what is the price decrease expressed as a percentage?

   A 30%

   B 36%

   C 47.5%

   D 37%

   E 37.5%

Example 2

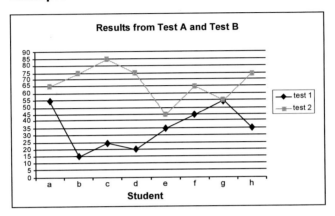

5   What was the overall average score for student 'f'?

  A   87

  B   55

  C   65

  D   76

  E   57

6   What was the median of the group's average score?

  A   40

  B   45

  C   55

  D   55.5

  E   56

7 **What was the mode of the group's average score?**

A   65

B   35

C   55

D   45

E   57

8 **What was the average pass mark of student 'a', expressed as a percentage, if both test scores were out of 90?**

A   69%

B   66.7%

C   64%

D   61%

E   63

Example 3

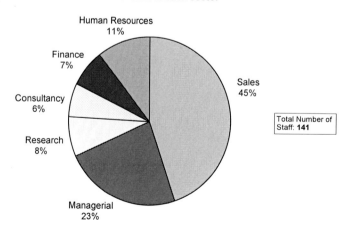

Number of staff in each sector

Human Resources 11%

Finance 7%

Consultancy 6%

Research 8%

Managerial 23%

Sales 45%

Total Number of Staff: **141**

14 There are 37.5 calories in a block of cheese, how much does the cheese weigh?

A   15 grams

B   16.6 grams

C   15.8 grams

D   16.9 grams

E   15.6 grams

15 How many calories are there in a 30 gram jam tart, which has a 23% reduction in calories?

A   32 calories

B   40 calories

C   48 calories

D   37 calories

E   39 calories

16 How many calories are there in 30 grams of butter, which has an 18% increase in calories?

A   212 calories

B   180 calories

C   212.4 calories

D   180.9 calories

E   232.7 calories

Example 5

Use the rates of exchange given in the table:

Country	Rate of Exchange
Europe (Euro)	€1.23 = £1.00
France (Franc)	Fr 10.8 = £1.00
Germany (Mark)	DM 3.4 = £1.00
Italy (Lire)	Lire 2600 = £1.00
Spain (Peseta)	Ptas 263 = £1.00
United States (Dollar)	$1.45 = £1.00

17 How many French Francs are you able to purchase with £20.00?

- A   216 Francs
- B   217 Francs
- C   817 Francs
- D   891 Francs
- E   206 Francs

18 How much is 6767 Euros worth in Pounds Sterling?

- A   £547.00
- B   £5501.63
- C   £5501.00
- D   £8323.41
- E   £5513.13

19 **A CD costs £22.00 in Britain and $15.00 in the United States. How much cheaper, in British currency, is the CD when brought in the USA?**

    A   £2.00

    B   £12.00

    C   £11.66

    D   £11.13

    E   £12.60

20 **A traveller in Switzerland exchanges 1500 Swiss Francs for £1200. What is the exchange rate?**

    A   2.23

    B   1.23

    C   1.25

    D   2.25

    E   1.50

Justification of Quantitative Reasoning practice examples

Example1

Question 1   **Answer D**

Step 1   We first need to find out the individual prices of the machines at wholesale. We do this by dividing the total price of 13 Brand G machines by the number of machines (13) therefore the calculation is:

£9843 ÷ 13 = £757.15 per machine

Step 2   We find the total of 11 Brand G machines at wholesale price, which is:

11 x £757.15 = £8328.65

Step 3   We then find the total of the machines sold at RRP, which is:

£923.40 x 11 = £10157.40

Step 4   We then find the difference between the total sold at the RRP and the total paid for the machines at the wholesale price, which is:

£10157.40 – £8328.65 = £1828.75 (Profit made)

Example 3

Question 9   **Answer E**

In order to find out the number of staff in each sector, we need to divide the percentage of staff by 100, then multiply this by the total number of staff working at the organisation. The following calculation determines the number of staff there are within the Human Resources sector.

(Percentage of staff in each sector) ÷ 100 x total number of staff

11% of the staff from the organisation are in the Human Resources sector.

(11 ÷ 100) x 141 = 15.51 (We then round this number to the nearest whole number) = 16

Question 10   **Answer D**

As explained above, we use the following formula for each of the sectors and combine them individually to find a total of 40 staff.

(Percentage of staff in each sector) ÷ 100 x total number of staff

Therefore there are 32 members of staff in the Management sector and 8 members of staff in the Consultancy sector; this leaves us with a total of 40 members.

Question 11   **Answer D**

Step 1   We first carry out the above formula and find out how many staff there are in each sector.

In the Sales division there are 63 staff members, and in the Managerial sector there are 32 staff members.

Step 2   We work out the difference between the total staff members in the Sales division and the Managerial sector:

63 – 32 = 31

Step 3   We take this difference and divide it by the combined total of staff members in both sectors, and then multiply this by 100 to get a percentage.

(31 ÷ 95) x 100 = 32.63%

Question 12   **Answer A**

(Percentage of staff in each sector) ÷ 100 x total number of staff

We take the above formula and work out how many members of staff there are in each sector. 8% of 141 staff are in the Research sector.

(8 ÷ 100) x 141 = 11 members of staff (To the nearest whole number)

Example 4

Question 13   **Answer C**

This requires a simple multiplication: in one gram of bread there are 1.2 calories. We then carry out the following calculation:

1.2 x 89 grams = 106.8 calories

Question 14   **Answer A**

This requires a simple division: total calories ÷ calories per gram of cheese = grams of cheese

37.5 ÷ 2.5 = 15 grams of cheese

Question 15   **Answer D**

Step 1

First we need to determine how many calories there are in the 30 gram jam tart: 1 gram of jam tart has 1.6 calories, therefore 30 grams of jam tart will have 48 calories.

30 grams of jam tart x 1.6 Calories = 48 calories

Step 2

Secondly, this particular jam tart has a 23% reduction in calories, hence we calculate a percentage decrease:

23% ÷ 100 x 48 = 11.04 calorie reduction

Step 3

We then subtract this calorie reduction from the original calories contained in the jam tart:

**48 – 11.04 = 37.0 calories
(1 decimal place)**

Question 16   **Answer C**

The previous question required the calculation of a percentage decrease; this question requires a percentage increase. We still use the same formula, although we then add the percentage increase to the final total:

Step 1   Determine how many calories there are in 30 grams of butter:

30 x 6 = 180 calories

Step 2   We now determine 18% of 180:

(18 ÷ 100) x 180 = 32.4

Step 3   We now add the 18% of 180 (32.4) to the final calorie intake:

32.4 + 180 = 212.4 calories

Example 5

Question 17   **Answer A**

This question requires a simple multiplication.

We simply multiply £20.00 by the rate of exchange (in this case it is French Francs and the exchange rate is 10.8):

20.00 x 10.8 = 216 Fr

Question 18   **Answer B**

This question requires the opposite calculation to the previous question, instead of multiplying we *divide* by the exchange rate:

6767 Euros ÷ 1.23 = £5501.63

Abstract Reasoning tests are usually presented in sequences and patterns, which involve symbols and shapes.

When attempting such questions, we need to understand the following concepts:

- Symmetry – are the shapes in a symmetrical format?

- Number patterns – is there a common pattern in the sequence of numbers, e.g. 2, 4, 6, 8 and so on?

- Size – do the shapes vary in size?

- Shapes – are there specific shapes being used?

- Characteristics – are the symbols and shapes curved; do they have straight lines or angles?

- Rotation – are the shapes or symbols rotated clockwise or anti-clockwise?

- Direction – are the symbols or shapes in any specific direction i.e. are they aligned diagonally, horizontally or vertically?

- Lines – are they continuous or dashed?

The Abstract Reasoning subtest consists of thirteen stems. Each stem comprises of two sets (Set A and Set B) which each contain six shape formations. You will then be presented with five further shape options which are the lead-in questions. You will be expected to identify whether each lead-in question belongs to either 'Set A', 'Set B' or 'Neither'.

You will be allocated a time limit of sixteen minutes for the Abstract Reasoning subtest which equates to approximately fifteen seconds for each answer. This time allocation includes one minute for administration purposes.

Summary of Abstract Reasoning structure

Stem

The stem will consist of a pair of shapes, these will be known as 'Set A' and 'Set B.' Each set will contain a total of six shapes, all which will have common themes. There will be a total of thirteen stems.

Lead-in question

For each stem there will be a total of five shapes which act as the lead-in questions. There will be a total of sixty-five lead-in questions.

Choices

Your task will be to decide whether the test shapes are part of 'Set A' or 'Set B' or 'Neither'.

Only one of the choices will be correct.

Time limit = sixteen minutes. Therefore you will have approximately fifteen seconds per question

When you are working through the UKCAT subtests it can be counter-productive to monitor exactly how long you spend on answering each question, especially when you need to read through and digest the information presented in the stem. Therefore a more useful time management approach is to divide each subtest into four quarters. So, in the case of the Abstract Reasoning subtest, after approximately four minutes you should be working on the fourth stem, after approximately eight minutes you should be commencing the seventh stem and so on. If you find yourself falling behind at these points you know that you need to pick up the pace.

Example of an Abstract Reasoning question

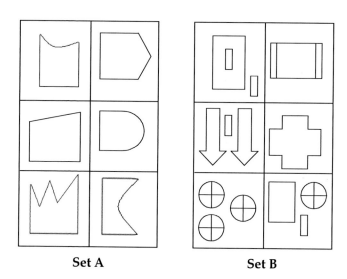

Set A   **Set B**

Test Shape 1

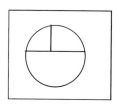

Answer: Set A, Set B or Neither

Abstract Reasoning hints and tips

Throughout the Abstract Reasoning subtest the shapes can be ordered in a variety of ways. The various patterns that can be used to distinguish between the shapes include:

- Symmetry – are the shapes symmetrical?

- Number patterns – is there a common pattern in the sequence of numbers, e.g. 2, 4, 6, 8 and so on?

- Size – do the shapes vary in size?

- Shapes – are there specific shapes being used?

- Characteristics – are the symbols and shapes curved; do they posses straight lines or angles?

- Rotation – are the shapes or symbols rotated clockwise or anti-clockwise?

- Direction – are the symbols or shapes in any specific direction i.e. are they aligned diagonally, horizontally or vertically?

- Lines of shapes – are they continuous, dashed or double lines?

Symmetrical Characteristics

- Some of the larger symmetrical shapes may be replicated amongst smaller '*distracter*' shapes.

- Some shapes may seem symmetrical at first glance but are in fact asymmetrical, such as a parallelogram.

- Some sets contain shapes which are symmetrical and are only made up of straight lines while asymmetrical shapes may be curved or vice versa.

- Some symmetrical shapes may have a dotted or dashed outline, asymmetrical shapes may have a solid outline or vice versa.

- Some sets may have symmetrical shapes which are shaded in black, while asymmetrical shapes may be white or vice versa.

Number patterns

- Certain number patterns may be symbolised by specific shapes. For example, if a set contained shapes in sets of 2, 4 and 6 they may be represented by small triangles.

- Some number patterns are often replicated in both sets; however the accommodating shapes may differ from one set to another. For example, in Set A, if there are small triangles in groups of 2, 4 and 6 and small circles in groups of 3, 6 and 9, this pattern may be reversed in Set B whereby there will be small circles in groups of 2, 4 and 6 and small triangles in groups of 3, 6 and 9.

- Some number patterns may be represented with various types of shading, e.g. black or white shading or different outlines e.g. dotted, dashed or solid outlines.

Size

- Do the shapes vary in size?
- Are certain sized shapes positioned in specific areas in a set?

- Often the same sized shapes are used in both sets, although they are positioned differently.

  For example in Set A, there could be three different sized circular shapes – small, medium and large. The smallest shape could always be positioned within the largest shape. The same sized shapes may also be used in Set B, however the rules change slightly and instead the medium sized circular shape could be positioned within the largest shape.

- Shapes may be shaded or un-shaded, for example curved shapes are shaded in black and shapes with straight lines are left white.

Characteristics

- Some sets may contain curved or straight lined shapes.

- A common method of causing confusion is to combine a mixture of curved and straight lines within a shape.

- Other sets may contain shapes which possess a dashed or solid outline or even a mixture of both.

- Some shapes may be present in differing quantities.

Rotation and direction

- Shapes can be positioned horizontally or vertically, and towards the middle, top, bottom, right or left of the test box.

- Shapes can be positioned in either a clockwise or anti-clockwise position.

3 simple steps to Abstract Reasoning

Once you acknowledge the various ways in which the shapes can be presented, you will find it easier to apply this knowledge if you follow the three simple steps below:

Step 1

First identify the different shapes and symbols used within each stem. Look for characteristics such as size, number and colour.

Step 2

Try to identify any patterns which the shapes or symbols form, such as reoccurring number patterns, rotation and positioning of shapes, symmetry and direction of shapes.

Step 3

Then try to identify the next part of the sequence for each lead-in question, and relate them to either 'Set A', 'Set B' or 'Neither'. If you really are unsure of the answer go with your gut instinct rather than leaving a blank.

Below you will find some examples of the types of Abstract Reasoning questions you will face when you attempt the UKCAT.

Abstract Reasoning practice examples
Example 1

Set A   **Set B**

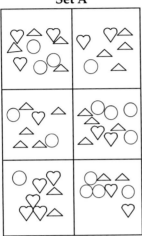
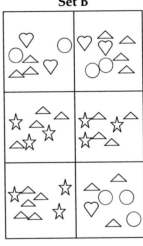

Test Shape 1

Set A

Set B

Neither

Test Shape 2

Set A

Set B

Neither

Test Shape 3

Set A

Set B

Neither

Test Shape 4

Set A

Set B

Neither

Test Shape 5

Set A

Set B

Neither

Example 2

Set A

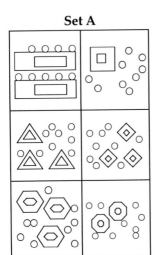

Set B

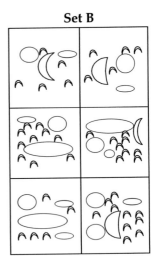

Test Shape 1

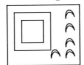

Set A

Set B

Neither

Test Shape 2

Set A

Set B

Neither

Test Shape 3

Set A

Set B

Neither

Test Shape 4

Set A

Set B

Neither

Test Shape 5

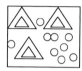

Set A

Set B

Neither

Example 3

Set A	Set B
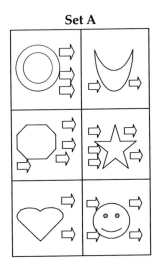	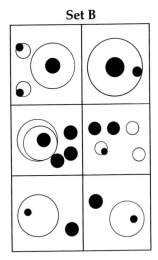

Test Shape 1

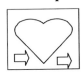

Set A

Set B

Neither

Test Shape 2

Set A

Set B

Neither

Test Shape 3

Set A

Set B

Neither

Test Shape 4

Set A

Set B

Neither

Test Shape 5

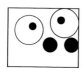

Set A

Set B

Neither

Example 4

Set A

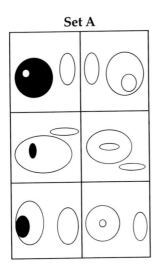

Set B

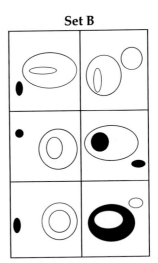

Test Shape 1

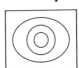

Set A

Set B

Neither

Test Shape 2

Set A

Set B

Neither

Test Shape 3

Set A

Set B

Neither

Test Shape 4

Set A

Set B

Neither

Test Shape 5

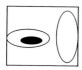

Set A

Set B

Neither

Example 5

Set A   **Set B**

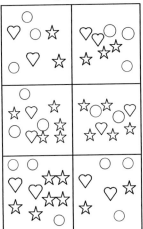 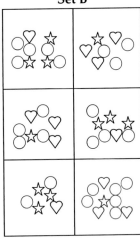

Test Shape 1

Set A

Set B

Neither

Test Shape 2

Set A

Set B

Neither

Test Shape 3

Set A

Set B

Neither

Test Shape 4

Set A

Set B

Neither

Test Shape 5

Set A

Set B

Neither

Example 6

Set A	Set B

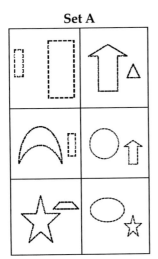
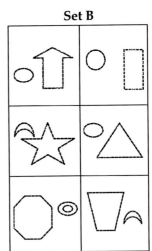

Test Shape 1

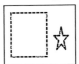

Set A

Set B

Neither

Test Shape 2

Set A

Set B

Neither

Test Shape 3

Set A

Set B

Neither

Test Shape 4

Set A

Set B

Neither

Test Shape 5

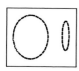

Set A

Set B

Neither

Example 7

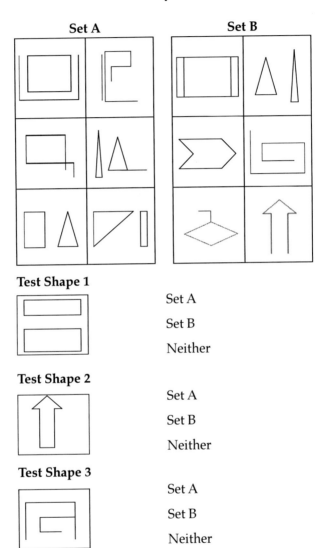

Set A   **Set B**

Test Shape 1

Set A

Set B

Neither

Test Shape 2

Set A

Set B

Neither

Test Shape 3

Set A

Set B

Neither

Test Shape 4

Set A

Set B

Neither

Test Shape 5

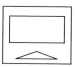

Set A

Set B

Neither

Justification of Abstract Reasoning practice questions

Example 1

Set A

- There are circular, heart and triangular shapes present.

- Collectively the circular and the heart shapes can be grouped into sets of three, six, and nine shapes. For example three heart shapes and three circular shapes or four circular shapes and five heart shapes.

- The triangles are used as distracters.

Set B

- There are heart, circular, triangular and star shapes present. The heart and circular shapes are always arranged together in groups of four. For example, two heart shapes and two circular shapes or one heart shape and three circular shapes.

- The star shapes are arranged in groups of three but are only in present in three of the boxes.

- The pattern to identify in Set B is slightly more complicated than Set A. The patterns are either heart or circular shapes collectively forming a group of four, or three star shapes present.

- The triangles have again been used as distracters.

Test Shape 1 – Neither

The shape arrangement comprises four hearts and five triangles. This therefore does not follow the above patterns for either set.

Test Shape 2 – Set A

There are three circular and three heart shapes present. Therefore this test shape follows the rules of Set A. This shape cannot belong in Set B as these particular shapes must be arranged in a group of four.

Test Shape 3 – Neither

This test shape comprises of four stars together with nine triangles which are used as distracters. The test shape looks similar to the pattern in Set B, but it does not follow the rule of three stars, instead it contains four stars.

Test Shape 4 – Set B

This test shape comprises two heart and two circular shapes, therefore it belongs to Set B as this pattern is not present in Set A. There are seven triangles but these act as distracters.

Test Shape 5 – Set B

The test shape has three stars with eight triangles used as distracters – this pattern is only present in Set B.

Example 2

Set A

- In each of the six boxes the pattern present is nine small circles together with randomly assigned symmetrical shapes which exhibit various angles.

- Each symmetrical shape has an identical but smaller shape present within its core.

- The key pattern in this set is to have a symmetrical shape with a smaller identical shape within its core.

- The second rule to note is that there are nine smaller circular shapes present in each box.

Set B

- There are either five or ten small crescent shapes present in each box.

- All the shapes used in this set have curved sides.

- The distracters used in this set are large curved shapes, which comprise a combination of circular, large crescent and various sized ovals shapes.

Test Shape 1 – Neither

The test shape comprises five small crescent shapes together with a large square. Inside the large square is another smaller square. This shape has incorporated patterns from both of the sets and is therefore similar to 'Neither'.

Test Shape 2 – Set B

The test shape comprises of nine miniature crescent shapes together with two larger crescent shapes and one oval shape. Therefore it follows the pattern of Set B.

Test Shape 3 – Neither

The test shape comprises two identical rectangles, with smaller rectangles contained inside them. However, there are only five small circular shapes present; therefore it does not follow the rules of Set A. The test shape therefore does not conform to either pattern.

Test Shape 4 – Neither

The test shape first appears to belong to Set B as there are three medium sized curved shapes. However, there are only nine small crescent shapes instead of either five or ten, therefore the rules of Set B are not followed.

Test Shape 5 – Set A

There are three symmetrical triangles with smaller triangles inside them. There are also nine smaller circles. Therefore the rules of Set A are followed.

Example 3

Set A

- Each box contains a large symmetrical shape.
- Each box contains various numbers of arrows.
- The arrows all point to the right.

Set B

- There are either three or six circular shapes present.
- The shapes comprise variously sized circles.
- The shapes are either shaded or un-shaded.
- The smallest and shaded circular shape is always present within a larger shape but never outside.

Test Shape 1 – Neither

This test shape looks closer to Set B, but it does not follow the rules of the set. There is only one large circle with a shaded circle inside it, instead of there being either three or six circular shapes present.

Test Shape 2 – Neither

The test shape is closest again to Set B, but if a small and shaded circular shape is present it must be contained within a larger shape. In this test shape, the smallest, shaded circular shape is outside of the larger circle.

Test Shape 3 – Set A

This test shape comprises a large symmetrical heart shape together with two arrows of the same size pointing to the right.

Test Shape 4 – Set A

This test shape comprises an oval shape together with three arrows of the same size pointing to the right.

Test Shape 5 – Set B

There are six circular shapes present. The two small circular shapes are present within larger un-shaded circular shapes.

Example 4

Set A

- There are always three shapes present in each box.

- There are three different sized circular or oval shapes which can be small, medium or large.

- The rule in this set is that the smallest circular or oval shape is always within the largest circular or oval shape.

- No other shape(s) should be present within each other.

- The shading is used as a distracter.

Set B

- There are always three shapes present in each box.

- Similar to Set A, there are three different sized circular or oval shapes which can be small, medium or large.

- The rule in this set is that the medium sized circular or oval shape is always within the largest circular or oval shape.

- No other shape(s) should be present within each other.

- The shading is used as a distracter.

Test Shape 1 – Set A

The test shape belongs to Set A as the smallest shape is within the largest shape, and there are three circular/oval shapes present.

Test Shape 2 – Neither

The test shape does not belong to either set as there are two shapes which are of the same shape and size. There are not three different sized circular shapes present.

Test Shape 3 – Neither

The test shape does not belong to either set as both the small and medium sized shapes are within the largest shape. Therefore this test shape tends to combine the rules of both sets.

Test Shape 4 – Set B

The medium sized shape is within the larger circular/oval shape.

Test Shape 5 – Neither

The test shape cannot belong to either set as the smallest shape is within the medium sized shape. Therefore it does not incorporate the large shape which is a requirement of both sets.

Example 5

Set A

The test shapes include heart, circular and star shapes. The rules for this set are as follows:

- Where there are two hearts there should be three circle shapes.
- Where there are three hearts there should be two circle shapes.
- The stars are used as distracters.

Set B

- The test shapes include heart, circular and star shapes.
- Where there is one heart there should be three star shapes.
- Where there are three hearts there should be one star shape.
- The circles are used as distracters.

Test Shape 1 – Neither

The test shape ignores the rules of both Set A and Set B. There is one heart shape and two star shapes as opposed to the three star shapes in Set B. It also does not follow the rules of Set A, as the heart shapes must appear in pairs.

Test Shape 2 – Set B

There are three heart shapes and one star shape present in accordance with the pattern in Set B. The circular shapes are used as distracters. The circular shapes cannot be related to Set A as they must be present in a pair together with a pair of heart shapes.

Test Shape 3 – Set A

There are two heart shapes and three circular shapes therefore the rules of Set A are followed.

Test Shape 4 – Set B

There are three star shapes with one heart shape which is consistent with the pattern in Set B. The test shape cannot belong to Set A, as it does not follow the rule of a pair of hearts in combination with a pair of circles.

Test Shape 5 – Neither

The test shape looks similar to Set B as there are three star shapes to one heart shape. However it does not follow the pattern of also containing circular shapes in the background.

Example 6

Set A

- In this set there are large straight and curved symmetrical shapes.

- The main rule for this set is that each shape must have a smaller corresponding symmetrical shape which is made of straight lines only.

Set B

- In this set there are large symmetrical shapes made only from straight lines.

- The main rule for this set is that each shape must have a smaller corresponding symmetrical shape which is made of curved lines only.

Test Shape 1 – Set A

The smaller shape is made of straight lines, and for this reason it belongs to Set A. It cannot be related to Set B as the smaller shape would have to be of a curved nature.

Test Shape 2 – Neither

The large shape is a parallelogram and is therefore not symmetrical. It cannot belong to either set.

Test Shape 3 – Set A

The smaller shape is made of straight lines, and therefore belongs to Set A. It cannot belong to Set B for two reasons; firstly, the smaller shape would need to have curved lines and secondly, the large shape can only be made of straight lines.

Test Shape 4 – Set B

The smaller shape is curved and hence belongs to Set B.

Test Shape 5 – Neither

The smaller shape is curved, which is a characteristic of Set B. However, the test shape cannot belong to Set B, as the large shape is also curved and this set only has large shapes made of straight lines.

Example 7

Set A

- The shapes present in each box comprise a maximum of seven sides.

Set B

- The shapes present in each box comprise a maximum of six sides.

Test Shape 1 – Neither

The test shape cannot belong to either set as there are a total of eight lines rather than seven or six lines.

Test Shape 2 – Set A

The test shape comprises of seven lines so the answer is Set A.

Test Shape 3 – Set B

The test shape belongs to Set B as the shape comprises a total of six lines.

Test Shape 4 – Set B

As above, the test shape belongs to Set B as it comprises a total of six lines.

Test Shape 5 – Set A

The test shape belongs to Set A as it comprises a total of seven lines.

Chapter 6

The Decision Analysis Subtest

The Decision Analysis test measures a candidate's ability to translate and make sense of coded information. This type of test measures a candidate's quality of decision making, in terms of accuracy, adequacy and the time taken in which the decision is made. Individuals must possess an exceptional ability to translate and identify related information, separate facts from fiction and consider all issues they are presented with. Achieving a high score in the Decision Analysis subtest reflects a candidate's ability to make decisions in real-life situations where the information provided is complex and from various sources.

The UKCAT Decision Analysis subtest consists of one scenario and twenty-six related items which form the basis of questions asked. The scenario itself may contain a table, text and various other sources of information and codes. You will be requested to interpret information given in the questions using the facts provided in the scenario.

You will find at times that the information which you have is either incomplete, or that it does not make sense. You will need to then make your best judgment based on the codes, rather than what you expect to see or what you think is reasonable. **Ensure that you base your decisions solely on the information provided to you.** There will always be a best answer which makes the most sense based on all the information presented. It is important that you understand that this test is based on judgements rather than simply applying rules and logic.

The Decision Analysis subtest differs from the other UKCAT subtests in that there can be more than five answer options for each question. Another notable difference from the other subtests is that candidates may be asked to give more than one response for a particular question. However, if this is the case then this will always be clearly stated within the question. You will have a time limit of thirty minutes for this section, which includes one minute for administration purposes, to answer twenty-six questions equating to just over one minute per question.

Summary of Decision Analysis structure

Stem

In this subtest you will be presented with one scenario comprising various facts and information, including codes.

Lead-in question

There will be twenty-six individual lead-in questions, based on just the one scenario (the stem).

Choices

For each of the lead-in questions you will be given a choice of five or more answers. These will be represented as A, B, C, D or E etc. In the previous subtests there was always only one correct answer. In this subtest you may be given the option of choosing more than one correct answer. This will always be clearly indicated in the lead-in question.

Time limit = thirty minutes. Therefore you will have sixty-nine seconds per question.

When you are working through the UKCAT subtests it can be counter-productive to monitor exactly how long you spend on answering each question, especially when you need to read through and digest the information presented in the stem. Therefore a more useful time management approach is to divide each subtest into four quarters. So, in the case of the Decision Analysis subtest, after approximately seven and half minutes you should be working on the seventh question, after approximately thirteen minutes you should be commencing the fourteenth question and so on. If you find yourself falling behind at these points you know that you need to pick up the pace.

Example of Decision Analysis question

Scenario (Stem)

A group of archaeologists have discovered a hidden pyramid. They have identified hieroglyphics on the walls which show various codes. The team have managed to decode some of the messages; these are presented in the table below. Your task is to examine particular codes or sentences and then choose the best interpretation of the code from one of five possible choices.

You will find, at times, that the information which you have is either incomplete or does not make sense. You will need to then make your best judgment based on the codes, rather than what you expect to see or what you think is reasonable. There will always be a best answer which makes the most sense based on all the information presented. It is important that you understand that this test is based on judgements rather than simply applying rules and logic.

Operating Codes	Basic Codes	Verbs
1 = Antonym	A = Sea	♎ = Dining
2 = Present	B = Oxygen	⊠ = Drinking
3 = Past	C = Person	♑ = Brawling
4 = Future	D = Sun	☐ = Seeing
5 = Increase	E = Night	♌ = Conversing
6 = Unite	F = Cold	☺ = Listening
7 = Plural	G = Today	♱ = Smiling
8 = Attribute	H = Tomorrow	∉ = Trusting
9 = Conditional	I = Weapon	
10 = Open	J = Creature	
11 = Positive	K = Hazard	
12 = Weak	L = She	
13 = Frequently	M = Run	
	N = Emotion	
	O = Building	
	P = Drop	
	Q = Jungle	
	R = Escape	
	S = Triumph	
	T = Move	

Lead-in question:

Examine the following coded message:
(A, 8), (7, C), O, 2

Now examine the following sentences and try to determine the most likely interpretation of the code.

Choices:

A People were behind the building near the river

B The church is across the lake

C People were in the building as they saw the attributes of the sea

D The community centre was across the lake

E The lake was near the church

Decision Analysis hints and tips

The following are common mistakes to look for when interpreting codes in a Decision Analysis subtest:

- **Various interpretations** of the same word can be used e.g. 'present', which could refer to time, as in 'the present moment', or otherwise to a gift, as in 'a birthday present'.

- Some of the answer options may include all of the encoded words but not make logical or grammatical sense.

- Some answer options **may not include all of the interpreted code words.**

- The interpreted words are **not necessarily in a specific order.** Therefore do not make the mistake of necessarily interpreting the codes in the exact order they are presented.

- **<u>Do not spend too long on a difficult question.</u>**
  Difficult questions are often easily identifiable
  by the length and complexity of the code
  – effective time management is key.

- Words within brackets are usually combined
  to give one meaning and should not be used as
  separate words within answer options.

- Certain codes require you to give your answer
  in a specific tense such as 'past', 'present' or
  'future'. These answers do not require you to
  actually state the word unless specified by other
  codes.

- Base your answer on the information provided
  – do not make subjective judgements.

- Where you are unable to distinguish between
  two answer options go with your gut feeling as
  this is normally correct.

- Use your whiteboard to make a note of the
  code interpretations as you work through each
  question to avoid confusion.

- You may be asked a question where you are
  provided with a line of text that you must
  convert into the correct code sequence.

3 simple steps to interpreting Decision Analysis questions

Step 1

Interpret the coded information given in the lead-in
question and write the words down on scrap paper

– remember to pay special attention to words in brackets.

Step 2

Translate the meaning of combined codes where applicable.

Step 3

Relate the words to each of the answer options; remember to take the following into account:

- Do the answer options make use of all of the words within the code?

- Which of the answer options are clearly incorrect or contain information not referred to in the scenario, and are therefore easy to eliminate?

- Do the answer options make use of the combined words and words in brackets correctly?

- Is the answer given in an order that reflects the code correctly and makes sense?

- Which answer options are clearly correct, and of these, which potential correct answer options arrive at the best interpretation of the code?

- An answer can still be correct if it does not contain the exact interpretation but is the best fit of all the answer options provided.

Decision Analysis practice example questions

Stem 1

An ancient ship has been discovered by a group of archaeologists. They have found a map and a letter which use various codes. The team have managed to decode some of the messages; these are presented in the table below. Your task is to examine particular codes or sentences and then choose the best interpretation of the code from one of five possible choices.

You will find, at times, that the information which you have is either incomplete or does not make sense. You will therefore need to make your best judgment based on the codes rather than what you expect to see or what you think is reasonable. There will always be a best answer which makes the most sense based on all the information presented. It is important that you understand that this test is based on judgements rather than simply applying rules and logic.

Operating Codes	Routine Codes
A = Opposite	1 = Sun
B = Decrease	2 = People
C = Negative	3 = Building
D = Cold	4 = City
	5 = Yesterday
	6 = Run
	7 = Sand
	8 = Danger
	9 = Tonight
	10 = Water
	11 = Tomorrow
	12 = Lonely
	13 = Anatomy
	14 = Head

Example 1

Examine the following coded message:

D, 9, (2, 12), 8

Now examine the following sentences and try to determine the most likely interpretation of the code.

A The cold will bring out dangerous people tonight

B It is cold tonight, and could be dangerous as there will be no one about

C Lonely people are dangerous tonight

D The dangerous cold will bring out lonely people tonight

E Lonely people are cold hearted

Example 2

Examine the following coded message:

(A, 8), 4, 2, (A, B)

Now examine the following sentences and try to determine the most likely interpretation of the code.

A It is safer in the city as there are more people

B The danger in the city is decreasing as there are people opposite

C The city has dangerous people

D The city has a decreased rate of dangerous people

E Opposite the city are dangerous men

New words have been added to the list. You may find that some of the codes are incomplete. However, you are asked to make your best judgement and not to answer on the basis of what you might consider being reasonable.

Operating Codes	Routine Codes	Specialist Codes
A = Opposite	1 = Sun	ℋ = Happy
B = Decrease	2 = People	❑ = Angry
C = Negative	3 = Building	◆ = Shy
D = Cold	4 = City	
	5 = Yesterday	
	6 = Run	
	7 = Sand	
	8 = Danger	
	9 = Tonight	
	10 = Water	
	11 = Tomorrow	
	12 = Lonely	
	13 = Anatomy	
	14 = Head	

Example 3

Examine the following coded message:

(1, ℋ), (A, 2)

Now examine the following sentences and try to determine the most likely interpretation of the code.

A   The sun makes people happy

B   The sun makes me happy

C   People make the sun happy

D   Happy people like the sunshine

E   The sun is happily shining

Example 4

Examine the following coded message:

(❑, 2), (D, A), 14

Now examine the following sentences and try to determine the most likely interpretation of the code.

A Angry peoples' bodies always get cold

B Angry people are hot-headed

C People who are angry get a hot head

D Angry people have cold heads

E People are angry when they get a cold

Example 5

Examine the following coded message:

4, 8, 10, (A, B)

Now examine the following sentences and select two of the most likely interpretations of the code.

A The city was very dangerous as it had rained a lot

B The rain decreased a lot in the city

C Paris was very dangerous due to the floods

D The flood was very dangerous

E The flood in the city was dangerous

Example 6

Examine the following coded message:

(A, 2), (A, 11), (3, 2)

Now examine the following sentences and try to determine the most likely interpretation of the code.

A People will be at the church today

B I will go to church today

C I met people opposite the building today

D Opposite the building there will be people

E Today there will be people opposite the church

Example 7

Examine the following coded message:

(A, B), (A,D), (A,2), 3, ⚸

Now examine the following sentences and try to determine the two most likely interpretations of the code.

A I was unhappy as my house was very cold

B I feel warm and very content when I go to the office

C I feel very warm and happy inside my house

D I was very happy to see the cold igloo

E Opposite the house stood warm happy people

Example 8

Examine the following coded message:

(A, D), 4, (A, 11)

Now examine the following sentences and try to determine the most likely interpretation of the code.

A The city will be very cold tomorrow

B London will be very cold today

C London will be warm, tomorrow

D London will be very warm today

E London is warm today

Example 9

Examine the following coded message:

(A, B), (A, 2), (10, 8), ☐

Now examine the following sentences and try to determine the most likely interpretation of the code.

A I was very angry that the sea was dangerous

B They were angry that the flood was dangerous

C The waves crashed very angrily

D I was very angry at the sight of the flood

E People were very angry at the sight of the rain

Example 10

Examine the following coded message:

(C, ⅝), (A, 2), ◆

Now examine the following sentences and try to determine the two of the most likely interpretations of the code.

A   I pretend to be happy when I am shy

B   I feel unhappy when I am shy

C   People feel both shy and happy

D   I was happy to see others shy

E   I feel negative towards other people as I am shy

Example 11

Examine the following sentence:

"I ran to the building as it was raining heavily"

Now examine the following codes and try to determine the most likely interpretation of the sentence.

A   (A, 2), 6, 3, 10

B   2, 6, 3, 10

C   10, (A, 2), 3

D   (A, 2), 3, (10, (A, B), 6

E   (A, 2), 6, 10

Example 12

Examine the following sentence:

"Her face had tears of happiness"

Now examine the following codes and try to determine the most likely interpretation of the sentence.

A 2, 13, & 10

B (A, 2), ⚸, 10

C (10, ⚸), (A, 2), 14

D 10, 2, ⚸

E (A, 2), 10, ⚸

Example 13

Examine the following sentence:

"There was no-one in the office as it was sunny today"

Now examine the following codes and try to determine the most likely interpretation of the sentence.

A 9, 3, 1, C

B C, 2, 3, 1, A, 9

C 1, (A, 9), 3

D (C, 2), 3, 1, (A, 9)

E (C, 2), 3, (A, 9), 4

Justification of Decision Analysis practice answers

Example 1   Answer B

D, 9, (2, 12), 8

The code combines the words *'Cold', 'Tonight', '(People, Lonely)', 'Danger'*

Option A	Ignores the word 'Lonely', and also ignores the rule of the brackets combining the words together.
Option B	**Is the correct answer as it uses all the codes. The words 'People' and 'Lonely' are combined, which can be interpreted as meaning "No-one".**
Option C	Incorporates the rule of combining the words 'People' and 'Lonely', however it still ignores the word 'Cold'.
Option D	Contains all of the words; however it does not flow logically.
Option E	Introduces the word 'Hearted', but it also ignores the words 'Danger' and 'Tonight'.

Example 2   Answer A

(A, 8), 4, 2, (A, B)

The code combines the words *'(Opposite, Danger)', 'City', 'People', '(Opposite, Decrease)'*

Option A	**Is the correct response. It combines all the words together, and uses the rules in the brackets, whereby the opposite of 'Danger' becomes 'Safer', 'City' and 'People' remain as they are and the opposite of 'Decrease' is 'Increase', which can be incorporated into the sentence as a large amount of people.**
Option B	Is incorrect as it disregards the rules of the brackets; however it still uses all of the words.
Option C	Ignores the rules of the brackets and excludes the word 'Decrease'.
Option D	Ignores the rules of the brackets.
Option E	Ignores the rules of the brackets, excludes the word 'Decrease' and introduces the word 'Men'.

Example 3   Answer B

(1,)(), (A, 2)

The code combines the words '(*Sun, Happy)', '(Opposite, People)*'

Option A	Is incorrect, although it uses all the words, it disregards the rules of the brackets.
Option B	**Is the correct answer; this is because it uses all the words within the code. Together with this, this option uses the following rules; it combines the**

words in the brackets, whereby the
sun has a 'Happy' characteristic to
it, and secondly it uses the rule of
using the opposite of 'People' which
is 'Person', but this has been replaced
with 'Me'.

Option C | Is incorrect as it ignores the rules of the brackets as mentioned above and secondly does not flow logically.

Option D | Uses all the words; however it ignores the rules of the brackets as previously mentioned.

Option E | Ignores the rules of the brackets and does not reference the words 'Opposite' and 'People'.

Example 4   Answer B

(□, 2), (D, A) 14

The code combines the words *'(Angry, People)'*, *'(Cold, Opposite)'*, *'Head'*.

Option A | Is incorrect as it interprets 'Head' as 'Body', and secondly it ignores the rules of the brackets whereby '(Cold, Opposite)' should be 'Hot'.

Option B | **Is the correct answer; this is because it uses all the words within the code. As well as this, this option combines the words in the brackets, whereby 'Angry' and 'People' are combined and '(Cold, Opposite)' is 'Hot', which is related to the 'Head'.**

Option C	Uses all the words; however it does not flow logically
Option D	The word 'Hot' should be used instead of 'Cold'.
Option E	Ignores the word 'Head' and the rules of the brackets.

Example 5   Answer A & C

4, 8, 10, (A, B)

The code combines the words *'Danger', 'City', 'Water', '(Opposite, Decrease)'*

Options A & C	**Are the correct responses, as they incorporate all the words contained within the code. 'Rain' is used instead of 'Water', and 'A lot' is used instead of 'Opposite' to 'Decrease'. In option C, 'Paris' is used as a replacement for the word 'City' and 'Floods' is used as a replacement for 'Water'.**
Option B	Ignores the rules of the brackets for '(Opposite, Decrease)'.
Option D	Ignores the word 'City'.
Option E	Ignores the words '(Opposite, Decrease)'.

Example 6   Answer B

(A, 2), (A, 11), (3, 2)

The code combines *'(Opposite, People)'*, *'(Opposite, Tomorrow)'*, *'(Building, People)'*

Option A	Ignores the words '(Opposite, People)'.
Option B	**Is the correct answer as 'I' replaces the words '(Opposite, People)', 'Today' replaces the words '(Opposite, Tomorrow)' and finally 'Church' replaces the words '(Building, People)' or, in other words, the code represents the words '(Public, Building)'.**
Option C	Ignores the rules of the brackets and does not combine the meanings of 'People' and 'Building' together.
Option D	Ignores the words '(Opposite, People)' and '(Opposite, Tomorrow)'.
Option E	Ignores the words '(Opposite, People)'.

Example 7   Answers B & C

(A, B), (A, D), 2, 3,)(

The code combines the words *'(Opposite, Decrease)'*, *'(Opposite, Cold)'*, *'(Opposite, People)'*, *'Building'*, *'Happy'*.

Option A	Uses the word 'Unhappy' and ignores the words '(Opposite, Cold)'.

Options B & C Are the correct answers. 'Very' replaces the words '(Opposite, Decrease)', 'Warm' replaces the words '(Opposite, Cold)', 'I' replaces '(Opposite, People)', 'Content' replaces 'Happy' and finally 'House' and 'Office' replace the word 'Building'.

Option D   Ignores the rules of the brackets for '(Opposite, Cold)' and 'Increase'.

Option E   Ignores the words '(Opposite, People)'.

Example 8   Answer E

(A, D) 4, (A, 11)

The code combines the words *'(Opposite, Cold)'*, *'City'*, *'(Opposite, Tomorrow)'*.

Option A   Ignores the rules of the brackets for '(Opposite, Cold)' and '(Opposite, Tomorrow)'.

Option B   Ignores the words '(Opposite, Cold)' and introduces the word 'Very'.

Option C   Ignores the words in brackets '(Opposite, Tomorrow)'.

Option D   Introduces the word 'Very'.

Option E   Is the correct answer. The word 'London' replaces 'City', 'Warm' replaces the words '(Opposite, Cold)', and 'Today' replaces '(Opposite, Tomorrow)'.

Example 9   Answer A

(A, B), (A, 2), (10, 8), ▢

The code combines the words *'(Opposite, Decrease)'*, *'(Opposite, People)'*, *'(Water, Danger)'*, *'Angry'*.

Option A	**Is the correct response; it makes use of all the words within the code. 'Sea' is used to describe 'Water', the word 'Very' emphasises the words '(Opposite, Decrease)' and 'I' replaces '(Opposite, People)'.**
Option B	Ignores the words in brackets '(Opposite, People)'.
Option C	Ignores the words in brackets '(Opposite, People)'.
Option D	Introduces the word 'Sight'.
Option E	Ignores the words in brackets '(Opposite, People)', and introduces the word 'Sight'.

Example 10   Answer A

(C, ⨯), (A, 2), ◆

The code combines the words *'(Negative, Happy)'*, *'(Opposite, People)'*, *'Shy'*.

Option A	**Is the correct option. It uses the word 'Happy' in a negative context, whereby the individual pretends to be happy. 'I' replaces the words '(Opposite, People)'.**

Option B	This statement appears to be correct but upon closer analysis the word 'Unhappy' is used instead of making a negative association.
Option C	Ignores the negative association of the word 'Happy', and ignores the rules in brackets of '(Opposite, People)'.
Option D	Ignores the negative association of the word 'Happy', and uses it in a positive light.
Option E	Uses all of the words, but does not make logical sense.

Example 11   Answer D

(A, 2), 3, (10, (A, B), 6

The code combines the words '*(Opposite, People)*', '*Building*', '*(Water, (Opposite, Decrease)*', '*Run*'

Option A	Does not include codes which describe the word 'Heavily'.
Option B	Is incorrect, as it ignores the codes which describe the word 'Heavily' and uses the code which describes 'People' instead of describing the word 'I'.
Option C	Ignores codes which portray the words 'Ran' and 'Heavily'.
Option D	**Is the correct response. The codes are used in the following way: 'I (Opposite, People) ran (Run) to the building as it was raining (Water) heavily (Opposite, Decrease)'.**

Option E Does not mention any codes which describe the word 'Heavily' or 'Building'.

Example 12 Answer C

(10, ⚥), (A, 2), 13

The code combines the words '*(Water, Happy)*', '*(Opposite, People)*', '*Head*'

Option A Does not use codes which describe the word 'Happiness'.

Option B Ignores codes which describe the word 'Face'.

Option C **Is the correct option as all of the codes apply to the sentence in the following way: 'Her (Opposite, People), face (Head) had tears of happiness' (combination of the words Water and Happiness)'.**

Option D Ignores codes which describe the word 'Her' and the word 'Face'.

Option E Ignores codes which describe the word 'Face'.

Example 13 Answer D

(C, 2), 3, 1, (A, 9)

The code combines the words '*(Negative, People)*', '*Building*', '*Sun*', '*(Opposite, Tonight)*'

Option A	Uses the code which describes 'Tonight' instead of the word 'Today'.
Option B	Uses all of the appropriate codes but does not use brackets to give the correct answer.
Option C	Ignores the code to describe the words 'No-one'.
Option D	**Is the correct option as all of the codes apply to the sentence accurately: 'There was no-one (Negative, People) in the office (Building) as it was sunny (Sun) today (Opposite, Tonight)'.**
Option E	Does not contain a code which describes the word 'Sunny' and introduces a code for the word 'City'.

Chapter 7

The Non-Cognitive Analysis Subtest

The Non-Cognitive Analysis subtest identifies whether or not a candidate's personal profile matches their chosen career path. In general, the Non-Cognitive subtest is fairly similar to a personality test. The main purpose of this test is to establish whether or not a candidate will be happy and content within their career; whether they will be able to cope and manage with the daily pressures and constraints, from being a student to a newly qualified medical or dental professional.

The Non-Cognitive Analysis subtest aims to explore aspects of a person's character that are thought to remain stable throughout their lifetime. The individual's pattern of behaviour, thoughts, feelings and emotions are all important concepts. The Non-Cognitive Analysis subtest aims to explore the following aspects:

- Robustness
- Empathy
- Integrity
- Honesty

Format of the Non-Cognitive Analysis subtest

The four concepts above will be identified by a questionnaire format in the UKCAT. Some questions will depict scenarios where candidates will be asked to decide what to do according to their morals, values and opinions. It is important to note that there are **no preferred answers**, and hence no answer is right or wrong. Candidates will be asked to choose an answer based on a scoring system. The choices will be presented as a series of options and candidates will need to choose an option which they believe closely fits their values and beliefs.

Other questions will include statements or pairs of statements of various concepts. These questions are specifically designed to measure a candidate's behaviour, attitudes, experiences and reactions to feelings of stress and well-being. With each question or statement candidates will be asked to specify how strongly they agree or disagree.

It is important that you answer the questions as truthfully as possible, as this test is designed to identify the 'Real you'. In addition to this, it is vital that you do not answer the questions according to 'How you think you may want to be seen'. These specific types of test have a built-in mechanism which identifies inconsistencies in a candidate's answers. For example, some of the questions are purposely designed to assess the degree of honesty the questionnaire has been approached with. It is also essential that you acknowledge that not all candidates will receive the same questions, as they will be randomly selected from a larger set of possible questions.

The actual Non-Cognitive Analysis subtest will take you no longer than thirty minutes to complete. However it has not been stated by the UKCAT how many questions there are in total. Generally speaking the majority of personality questionnaires usually consist of approximately 100 to 150 items, in the given time limit. That said, it is only an estimate and hence you may find the number of items are actually less than the indicated estimate.

Illustrated below are examples of the types of questions you may find in the Non-Cognitive Analysis subtest. You may find it beneficial to work through these, in order to familiarise yourself with the content of this section of the UKCAT.

Summary of Non-Cognitive structure

This section of the UKCAT does not contain any 'Stem' specific questions. Instead there are various scenarios and statements which candidates are required to show their degree of agreement to.

Time limit = thirty minutes. There is no specific number of questions for this subtest.

Example 1

Tom, Lee and Joe are working together on a science experiment. Tom is tasked with recording the results while Lee and Joe carry out the experiment. After working on the experiment for a few hours, Lee notices that the information that Tom has written is incorrect. Lee tells Joe and they both realise they would have to start the whole experiment again. Lee suggests that they should tell Tom and get him off their group. However Joe suggests that would be an unfair decision. Instead Joe suggests that they should tell Tom that it is someone else's turn to do the recording of the results. Lee feels that they would be lying, but Joe replies that they would not be hurting anyone else's feelings.

What is your opinion? How do you feel about each of the following statements?

There is no harm in lying if we are protecting the feelings of others.

☐ Strongly Agree

☐ Agree

☐ Disagree

☐ Strongly Disagree

Lying is always wrong.

☐ Strongly Agree

☐ Agree

☐ Disagree

☐ Strongly Disagree

It is always important to achieve the best marks, whatever it takes.

☐ Strongly Agree

☐ Agree

☐ Disagree

☐ Strongly Disagree

The truth must be told, regardless of who gets hurt.

☐ Strongly Agree

☐ Agree

☐ Disagree

☐ Strongly Disagree

It is always important to achieve the best marks, whatever it takes.

☐   Strongly Agree

☐   Agree

☐   Disagree

☐   Strongly Disagree

Some achievements in life are more important than friendships.

☐   Strongly Agree

☐   Agree

☐   Disagree

☐   Strongly Disagree

A good friend will always tell the truth, be it good or bad.

☐   Strongly Agree

☐   Agree

☐   Disagree

☐   Strongly Disagree

Example 2

The following example contains statements about how you may behave in various situations and statements about how others behave. Read each of the statements carefully and quickly decide whether you think each statement is:

☐ Definitely True

☐ True on the whole

☐ False on the whole

☐ Definitely False

I know I am able to stick to deadlines under pressure.

☐ Definitely True

☐ True on the whole

☐ False on the whole

☐ Definitely False

My peers would describe me as a friendly and easy-going person.

☐ Definitely True

☐ True on the whole

☐ False on the whole

☐ Definitely False

I strive hard to overcome challenges and achieve

☐   Definitely True

☐   True on the whole

☐   False on the whole

☐   Definitely False

I have the ability to stick to deadlines whilst being under immense pressure.

☐   Definitely True

☐   True on the whole

☐   False on the whole

☐   Definitely False

I would rather follow the opinions of the majority of the group rather than put forward my differing perspectives.

☐   Definitely True

☐   True on the whole

☐   False on the whole

☐   Definitely False

Example 3

Another part of the subtest will include a section of paired statements which will represent opposing perspectives. Read the following statements and state your degree of agreement by ticking the box that satisfies your answer.

1.

☐   **I worry a lot about stressful work loads**
☐
☐
☐
☐
☐   **I do not worry a lot about stressful workloads**

2.

☐   **I start quarrels with others easily**
☐
☐
☐
☐
☐   **I do not start quarrels with others easily**

3.

☐ **I persevere until the task is finished**

☐

☐

☐

☐

☐ **I do not persevere until the task is finished**

4.

☐ **I adapt my behaviour to meet others'
expectations**

☐

☐

☐

☐

☐ **I never adapt my behaviour to meet others' the
expectations**

5.

☐ **I trust people easily**

☐

☐

☐

☐

☐ **I do not trust people easily**

Chapter 8

Entire Mock UKCAT Exam

We would recommend that you complete the mock test under timed conditions and that you do not look at the answers until you have completed the test. The mock test should be completed in 90 minutes.

You will need to print the answer sheet which is available to download for free from www.apply2.co.uk

PLEASE NOTE THERE IS NO NON-COGNITIVE SECTION IN THE MOCK TEST

Verbal Reasoning – 22 minutes

Question 1

> *It has been suggested that listening to music may develop an individual's imaginative ability. It can help people concentrate on thoughts, brainstorm ideas, help creativity in the formation of art and inventions and help people formulate solutions to complex tasks and theories. There have been examples of scientists who have exploited music to help them learn, give inspiration to introduce novel concepts and knowledge, and find solutions to complicated scientific notions. For example, Albert Einstein would often listen to a violin piece while deep in thought, trying to solve physics problems.*

A   Listening to music will enhance a scientist's creativity

B   If an individual listened to classical music, originality may be achieved

C   Einstein developed solutions to various problems by playing a violin

D   Listening to music will allow an individual to become more creative

Question 2

> *Copper is usually used for the voice coil, however other metallic elements such as aluminium can also be utilised. The voice coil wire can be circular, rectangular or even hexagonal. A range of various voice coil wires are used in order to give different*

> *volume coverage, within a magnetic gap. The voice coil is positioned coaxially inside the gap. This gap is in actual fact a small circular hole, within the magnetic structure in order for the voice coil to be able to move back and fourth. This gap creates a powerful magnetic field amid the poles of a permanent magnet, whereby the outside of the gap acts as a singular pole, and the centre post serves as the other. The centre post and the back plate are known as the 'Yoke'.*

A   Voice coil wires come in various geometrical shapes, such as circular in a two dimensional figure with five sides and five equal angles, or they can be a four sided plane figure with four right angles

B   The small circular hole creates a robust magnetic field outside the poles of a magnet

C   A pole is situated at the hub of the magnetic field; this is also known as the 'Yoke'

D   There is a physical magnet in the voice coil

Question 3

> *From October 2006, The Employment Equality (age) Regulations make it illegal to discriminate against workers, employers, jobseekers and trainees due to their age. Direct discrimination is set out in the regulations, and states that it is unlawful, on the grounds of age, to come to a decision about employing someone or dismissing someone, to refuse to provide training, to deny individuals promotion and to make individuals work in adverse conditions.*

> *The second form of discrimination (indirect discrimination) is related to selection criteria, benefits, policies, and various employment rules and practises which may disadvantage particular people of specific ages, unless the practise which is utilised is justified.*
>
> *The regulation also allows organisations to predetermine the retirement age of 65. This therefore means that one is able to set retirement ages at or above 65.*

A   A job vacancy specifically advertising for graduates is a form of discrimination

B   Indirect discrimination refers only to an organisation's guiding principals

C   The act will allow a 75 year old to be in employment

D   An organisation justifies that an 18 year old is unable to be considered as a candidate as he or she does not have the right qualifications. This is a form of age discrimination

Question 4

> *Applications are now being accepted for the following courses; advanced and foundation Danish, intermediate Ukrainian, advanced, intermediate and foundation Bulgarian, and finally intermediate and foundation Russian. All of the courses will include an Introductory Workshop, with the exception of the non European languages. You can pick up an application form from the Institute of Foreign Arts; applications will need to be submitted by 10th March 2007.*

> *A 10% deposit will need to be paid in advance before the commencement of the course and thereafter payments can be made in four quarterly instalments. By the fourth instalment the course will be completed.*

A The institution only teaches European languages

B The course lasts for a whole year

C The languages which the institute advertises courses for are all European

D The Institute of Foreign Arts has all the application forms

Question 5

> *Although autism was first discovered in 1943, it is still a relatively unknown disability. Children with autism do not show any signs of physical disability. It is a lifelong development disability that affects an individual's social interaction, social imagination and communication skills. Most sufferers can often have learning difficulties.*
>
> *A form of autism is called Asperger's syndrome, which is used to describe sufferers who are usually at the higher functioning end of the autistic spectrum. It seems that to an autistic person reality is a confusing, interacting mass of events, people, places, sounds, and sights. A sufferer may not have clear boundaries, order or meaning to anything.*

A People who see an autistic child may assume they look 'normal'

B Autistic children may not have the ability to develop reciprocal relationships

C Autistic children are unable to make sense of their world

D Autistic children are able to comprehend and put forward new ideas about creative play

Question 6

The legislative maternity privileges shape a minimum standard of protection recognised by Parliament. Women and their employers (or their legislative bodies) are able to negotiate and consent to more constructive provision on a voluntary or contractual foundation, if they feel that this would be more beneficial in the long term. Where an employer and employee have agreed diverse provisions, an employee will always be able to declare her statutory rights if these are better than those agreed with her employer, therefore if the employee wishes a term by maternity privileges she is able to do so. This therefore means that an employee will not be obliged to accept maternity arrangements which are not as good as the legislative rights.

In order to qualify for Statutory Maternity Pay, an employee will have to be an employed earner, therefore the employee will need to work for an organisation that is liable to pay the employee's share of National Insurance contributions.

To qualify for Maternity Allowance an employee must be, or have recently been either an employed or self-employed earner. The majority of people, who qualify for leave will also qualify for pay, and vice versa. All employees who are parents to new babies have a right to statutory leave with pay. However, there are a few legal clauses. For instance, the privileges relating to time off for antenatal care, to maternity leave and to protection against detriment or unfair dismissal in connection with maternity leave do not apply to the following groups: members of the police force, MPs, the judiciary and various company directors, or to masters or crew members engaged in share fishing paid solely by how much stock they have caught.

A   Women are entitled to all legislative maternity privileges

B   In order for an individual to qualify for maternity allowance, an employee will have to work for an organisation who are liable to pay the employee's share of National Insurance contributions

C   Men are allowed time off if they are a parent to a new baby

D   The rights described in the passage above only relate to employees, and not those who are unemployed

YOU ARE NOW OVER THE HALFWAY STAGE. IDEALLY YOU SHOULD HAVE APPROXIMATELY NINE MINUTES LEFT

(Please note this prompt will not be given in your actual test)

Question 7

> Healthcare workers are at an increased risk of both fatal and non fatal injuries, due to a number of various factors ranging from violence within the workplace to apparatus being placed carelessly such as syringes and needles. However, recent research has found that there has been a decrease in medical and mental healthcare, and instead there is a high increase in the use of hospitals for severely disturbed violent cases, severe mental illness, drug abuse, or other types of out-of-the-ordinary behaviours by some patients. This form of violence is increasing in severity and frequency, in areas such as pharmacies, hospitals and community care facilities, and has now become a seemingly never-ending problem. It has been proposed that a resolution to such a problem would be to restrict the premature discharge of the chronically mentally ill from professional care services.

A   Increased risk of injury to healthcare workers is wholly due to an increase in healthcare and a decrease in the hospitalisation of those with mental health problems

B   If hospitalised patients remain in specialist care for longer periods, a decrease in injuries may be seen

C   Individuals who show atypical behaviours have been shown to be hospitalised

D   All mentally ill patients show violent behaviours

Question 8

Marketing and advertising books via various internet sites is becoming most popular with traders. This is chiefly because it costs less to publicise the actual book, as compared to traditional methods such as conferences and advertisements on billboards and in newspapers. Books are also stored in large warehouses prior to being dispatched to customers, nationally and internationally. Therefore overheads are also less. Whilst this may be true, publishers feel that they are not gaining an adequate amount from book sales, and are not just demanding that they are paid for the cover prices of the books, but also that they receive a percentage of the actual amount received for them. However, these discounts only seem possible on books which are bestsellers.

A The consumer demand for books which are sold over the internet is increasing

B The general recurring costs of running a publishing business are high

C Internet bookstores tender the greatest concession on the least popular books

D Conventional methods of publicising a book are more expensive

Question 9

Cardiovascular Disease (CVD) cost the healthcare system around £14,750 million in 2003, which is a cost per person of just below £250. 76% of these costs went towards hospital healthcare and 18% can be accounted for by drugs and dispensing.

Coronary Heart disease (CHD) cost the healthcare system around £3,500 million in 2003, which is a cost per person of just below £60. 79% of these costs were put towards hospital care and 16% towards drugs and dispensing.

There are also non healthcare costs including those from 'Production losses' from death and illness in those who were in employment. Informal care of people with the disease greatly adds to the financial burden.

In 2003, CVD related production losses stood at £6,200 million due to mortality and morbidity, with approximately 60% of this cost specifically due to death and 40% due to illness in those of working age. The cost of informal care for people with CVD was just over £4,800 million in 2003.

In 2003, production losses due to mortality and morbidity associated with CHD cost over £3,100 million, with around 30% of this cost specifically due to death and 70% due to illness in those of working age, stalling by 10% when compared to previous costs in 2002. The cost of informal care for people with CHD was around £1,250 million in 2003.

A The overall healthcare system costs for CHD and CVD increased by at least 49.1% when compared to the overall production losses

B The per capita cost for CVD was relatively higher than the per capita cost for CHD

C There are a total of approximately 59 million patients on whom the CVD costs are based

D The production losses specifically due to death for CHD are higher than the production losses related to CVD

Question 10

The Scottish and Newcastle brewery have blamed the unpredictable weather for the drop in their profits for the year 2007. Statistics show last years net profits of £76 million had dropped by 9% in the first six months of this year compared to the same period the previous year. The wet weather has been prominent throughout summer and, due to the fact that there is no large sporting event such as the 2006 football World Cup to increase sales, this has led to a further 4.3% drop for the remainder of the year. The chairman of Scottish and Newcastle has claimed that the continuation of this bad weather in the UK and France will make it most challenging to reach this year's target.

The Fosters beer company introduced a new low calorie line in 2006 with the intention of inflating their profits. This inflated Fosters' profits by 55.5%. This figure is still rising today. While the profits for Fosters' low calorie beer continue to rise, the proportion of the original Fosters' profits were 50% of Scottish and Newcastle's previous net profits.

A Scottish and Newcastle's profits in 2007 were
£65.9 million

B The 'original' Fosters line profits for 2007 are
£38 million

C The breweries are suffering profit decrease due to
long periods of bad weather

D Fosters' profits from 2006 and 2007 are lower than
the profits Scottish and Newcastle breweries made
in 2006

Question 11

The Santa Monica is a well defined unit of transverse mountain ranges in Southern California, situated at the core of the island. These ranges are perpendicular to the coast of Sierra Nevada and the Pennsylvania ranges. A mile of pink blossom trees brightens the pathway of each peak. Santa Monica, or 'the high one' as it is known, is often hidden away in the heavens. On a winter's day, one can see only the barks of blossom trees. Each mountain top has a layer of snow like icing on a cake. The triple peaks glisten like diamonds in a river, beneath the sunshine over the heart of the coast. Opposite Santa Monica lies its twin, Santa Louisa with three snow-layered peaks. However, Santa Louisa still looks like a baby when compared to 'the high one'.

A Mount Santa Monica is to be found at the heart of the island

B The Mountain has an identical twin across the island

C Santa Monica is high enough to almost reach the sky

D The Santa Monica is at right angles to the coast of Sierra Nevada

Quantitative Reasoning – 20 minutes

Book Readership:

Book	Total Readership (Millions)		% breakdown of adults reading each book in 1998	
	1981	1998	Male Adults	Female Adults
A Warm Day	2.2	8.9	22	18
My Best Friend	2.9	6.6	4	3
The Darkness in the Mind	3.5	2.1	24	6
Alive in the Past	6.9	4.8	10	13

1 Which book was read by a higher percentage of females than males in 1998?

A A Warm Day

B My Best Friend

C The Darkness in the Mind

D Alive in the Past

E A Warm Day and My Best Friend

2 What was the combined readership of 'Alive in the Past', 'A Warm Day' and 'My Best Friend' in 1981?

A 11 million

B 12 million

C 13 million

D 11.2 million

E 12.5 million

3 What was the percentage decrease for readership of 'Alive in the Past' from 1981 to 1998?

A 30.43 %

B 30.23 %

C 2.1 %

D 32.9 %

E 32.1%

4 How many male adult readers read a 'A warm Day' in 1998?

A 89000000

B 1958000

C 1.958

D 8900

E 4895000

The table below shows the results of a test for pulse rate conducted on 274 children:

	Number of Boys	Number of Girls
High pulse	68	61
Low pulse	73	73
Total	141	133

5 What percentage of the boys had a low pulse rate?

A 51.8%

B 51.2%

C 59.3%

D 54.0%

E 50.8%

6 What percentage of the children had a high pulse rate?

A 57.1%

B 47.1%

C 57.0%

D 61.0%

E 50.2%

7 What percentage of the group were girls?

A 53.5%

B 45.5%

C 78.5%

D 24.5%

E 48.5%

8 What was the mode of the pulse rates recorded?

A Boys' high pulse rate

B Girls' high pulse rate

C Boys' low pulse rate

D Girls' low pulse rate

E Girls' and boys' low pulse rate

Below you will find a menu for a café:

Ciabbata with cheese and onion	£3.20
Jacket potato	£1.20
Fries	£1.00
Pizza slice	£2.00
Onion rings	£1.00
Sausage and mash potato	£2.39

9   What is the mean average of the prices? (To the nearest penny)

A £1.78

B £1.82

C £1.80

D £2.80

E £1.86

10 What is the median of the prices?

A £1.89

B £1.90

C £1.60

D £2.00

E £1.20

11 What is the range of the price list?

A £3.20

B £2.89

C £2.20

D £1.00

E £2.30

12 What is the total of the mean, the median and the range?

A £4.60

B £3.76

C £1.98

D £5.60

E £5.20

Carefully study the Pie chart below:

Pie chart showing the various sectors which graduate work in after leaving university

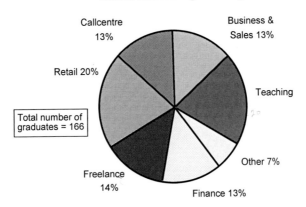

Total number of graduates = 166

13 How many graduates are there within the Teaching sector? (Round off to the nearest whole number)

A 30

B 23

C 31.2

D 34.9

E 33

14 How many more people are there in the Retail than the Freelance sector? (Round off to the nearest whole number)

A 10.2

B 10

C 11

D 15

E 9.1

15 Which two sectors have a total of 44 graduates? (Round off to the nearest whole number)

A Finance and Business & Sales

B Business & Sales and Teaching

C Finance and Freelance

D Teaching and Call Centre

E Freelance and Business & Sales

16 What is the ratio of those in the Teaching sector compared to those in the Retail sector?

A 33:33

B 3:3

C 1:1

D 11:22

E 34:34

Carefully study the line graph below and answer the following questions:

Production Number of 20cm Silver Chains

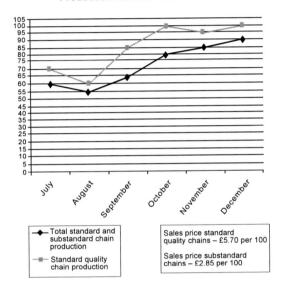

17 **What percentage of the total chain production was classed as substandard in September?**

A 13.5%

B 16.5%

C 17.5%

D 22.0 %

E 23.5%

18 By how much did the total sales value of chain production in November vary from October?

A   Decrease of £0.1425

B   Decrease of £1425.00

C   Increase of £25.00

D   No change

E   Increase of £5.00

19 What is the ratio of substandard to standard chains in October?

A   80:20

B   20:80

C   2:8

D   8:2

E   1:4

20 What was the percentage of substandard chains produced in July?

A   15.28

B   14.39

C   14.19

D   12.89

E   14.29

**THIS IS THE HALFWAY STAGE. IDEALLY YOU SHOULD HAVE APPROXIMATELY TWENTY MINUTES LEFT
(Please note this prompt will not be given in your actual test)**

Carefully study the bar chart below:

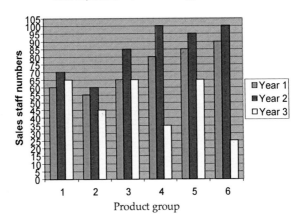

Sales department – Staff numbers, years 1 to 3

21 Which year had the greatest staff numbers?

A   Year 3

B   Year 2

C   Year 1

D   Can't tell

E   Year 4

22 What was the total number of staff in year 3?

A   200

B   300

C   350

D   240

E   500

23 What was the percentage decrease from year 1 to year 3, for the staff members in product group 4?

A 33.7%

B 23.9%

C 39.13%

D 45.75%

E 56.25

24 What is the mean for the total staff members in year 1?

A 72.1

B 78.2

C 72.5

D 79.5

E 74.0

Carefully study the table below:

Height of garage door (metres)	5 – 5.9	6 – 6.9	7 – 7.9	8 – 8.9	9 – 9.9
Number of garage doors	4	12	16	24	36

25 How many garage doors are ≤ 6.9 metres?

A 15

B 4

C 12

D 18

E 16

26 **Out of the total number of garage doors measured, how many are ≤ 7.9 meters? (Give your answer as a fraction of the total number).**

A 32/92

B 19/23

C 23/72

D 8/23

E 4/23

27 **What is the ratio of garage doors which are 6 – 6.9 metres to those which are 8 – 8.9 metres?**

A 12:36

B 36:12

C 1:2

D 6:2

E 12:24

28 **If 5 garage doors are each 12.9 metres high, what is their total height in centimetres (cm)?**

A 64.5 cm

B 645 cm

C 6450 cm

D 6.450 cm

E 6525 cm

Carefully study the table below:

Plumbers maintenance contract per month	Call out not under a maintenance contract
£150.00	£456.00

29 How many call outs per year would you have to make in order to make the maintenance contract worth paying the money?

A 3

B 2

C 4

D 3.17

E 5

30 If the plumber made a 25% profit on each call out not under a maintenance contract, how much profit does the plumber make on 12 call outs?

A £5472

B £1368

C £6840

D £5497

E £1656

31 How much would a maintenance contract cost for 3 years with a 12% discount?

A £648.00

B £5616.00

C £4567.00

D £4752.00

E £4942.08

Here is a recipe for making chocolate biscuits for 4 people:

Weight	Ingredient
689 grams	Self raising flour
100 grams	Sugar
124 grams	Margarine
256 grams	Chocolate

37 Bars of chocolate are sold in 200g blocks. How many bars would you need to buy to make biscuits for 11 people?

A 2 bars

B 3 bars

C 4 bars

D 5 bars

E 6 bars

38 If 1705 grams of margarine is used in the recipe, how many servings is this recipe now based on?

A 12

B 45

C 66

D 56

E 55

39 Of the total amount of ingredients contained in the recipe, what percentage of sugar is required? (Give your answer to 2 decimal places)

A 8.55%

B 8.14%

C 85.5%

D 11.25%

E 0.85%

40 What is the ratio of margarine to chocolate?

A 62:128

B 1:64

C 64:31

D 31:64

E 32:64

Abstract Reasoning – 16 minutes

Question 1

Set A   Set B

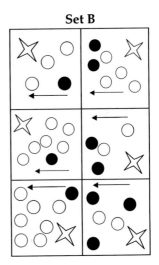

Test Shape 1

Test Shape 2

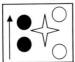

Test Shape 3

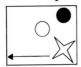

Test Shape 4

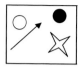

Test Shape 5

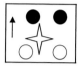

Question 2

Set A

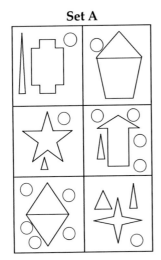

Set B

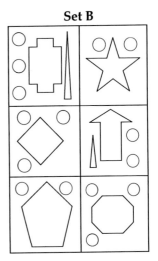

Test Shape 1

Test Shape 2

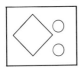

Test Shape 3

Test Shape 4

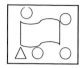

Test Shape 5

Question 3

Set A   Set B

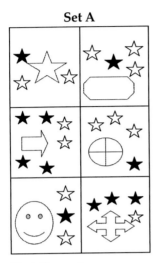 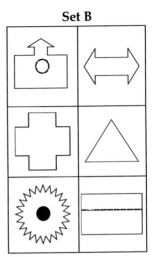

Test Shape 1

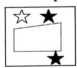

Test Shape 2

Test Shape 3

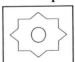

Test Shape 4

Test Shape 5

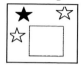

Question 4

Set A   Set B

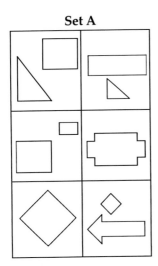 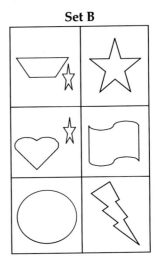

Test Shape 1

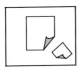

Test Shape 2

Test Shape 3

Test Shape 4

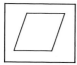

Test Shape 5

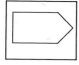

Question 5

Set A

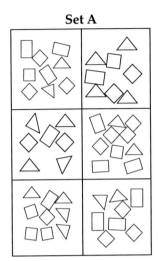

Set B

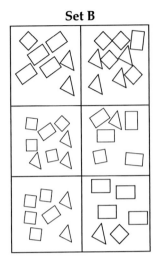

Test Shape 1

Test Shape 2

Test Shape 3

Test Shape 4

Test Shape 5

Question 6

Set A   **Set B**

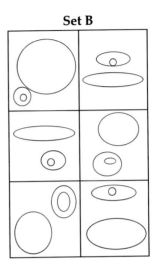

Test Shape 1

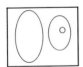

Test Shape 2

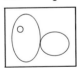

Test Shape 3

Test Shape 4

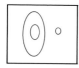

Test Shape 5

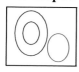

Question 7

Set A   Set B

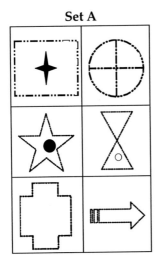   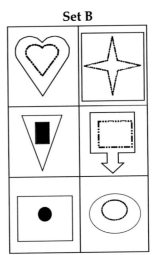

Test Shape 1

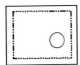

Test Shape 2

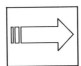

Test Shape 3

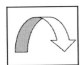

Test Shape 4

Test Shape 5

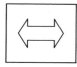

YOU ARE NOW OVER THE HALFWAY STAGE.
IDEALLY YOU SHOULD HAVE APPROXIMATELY
SEVEN MINUTES LEFT

(Please note this prompt will not be given in your
actual test)

Question 8

Set A	Set B

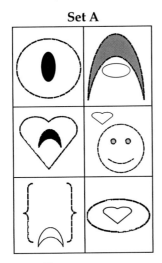
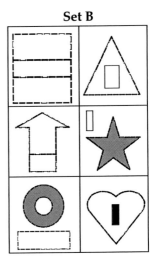

Test Shape 1

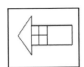

Test Shape 2

Test Shape 3

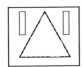

Test Shape 4

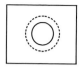

Test Shape 5

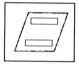

Question 9

Set A   **Set B**

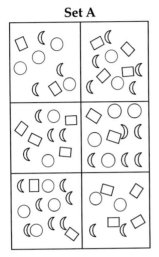   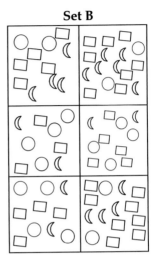

Test Shape 1

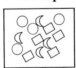

Test Shape 2

Test Shape 3

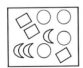

Test Shape 4

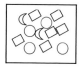

Test Shape 5

Question 10

Set A	Set B

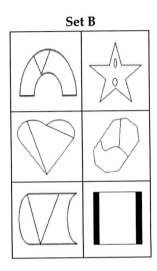

Test Shape 1

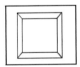

Test Shape 2

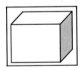

Test Shape 3

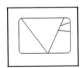

Test Shape 4

Test Shape 5

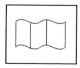

Question 11

Set A

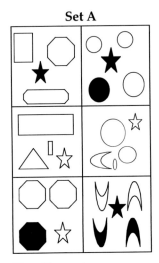

Set B

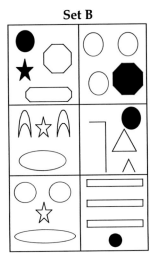

Test Shape 1

Test Shape 2

Test Shape 3

Test Shape 4

Test Shape 5

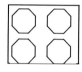

Question 12

Set A

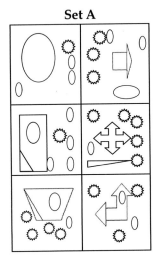

Set B

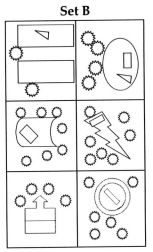

Test Shape 1

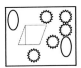

Test Shape 2

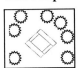

Test Shape 3

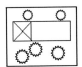

Test Shape 4

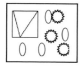

Test Shape 5

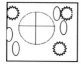

Question 13

Set A   Set B

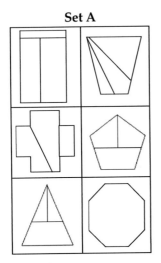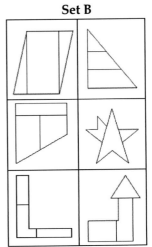

Test Shape 1

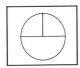

Test Shape 2

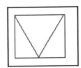

Test Shape 3

Test Shape 4

Test Shape 5

Decision Analysis – 30 minutes

A group of historians have discovered a cave with various paintings and symbols on the walls. The team have managed to decode some of the messages; these are presented in the table below. Your task is to examine particular codes or sentences and then choose the best interpretation of the code from one of five possible choices.

You will find, at times, that the information which you have is either incomplete or does not make sense. You will need to make your best judgment based on the codes rather than what you expect to see or what you think is reasonable. There will always be a best answer which makes the most sense based on all of the information presented. It is important that you understand that this test is based on judgements rather than simply applying rules and logic.

Operating Codes	Routine Codes	Specialist Codes
A = Opposite	1 = Sun	⧖ = Happy
B = Decrease	2 = People	☐ = Angry
C = Negative	3 = Building	◆ = Shy
D = Cold	4 = City	♒ = Assertive
E = Similar	5 = Yesterday	● = Intelligent
F = Disregard	6 = Run	○ = Extraverted
G = Quickly	7 = Sand	⚐ = Daring
H = Merge	8 = Danger	♋ = Trusting
I = Up	9 = Tonight	⌘ = Unstable
J = Weak	10 = Water	
K = Hard	11 = Tomorrow	
L = Desire	12 = Lonely	
	13 = Ice	
	14 = Sea	
	15 = Footprints	
	16 = Storm	
	17 = Light	
	18 = Anatomy	
	19 = He	
	20 = Structure	
	21 = Security	
	22 = Natural	
	23 = They	
	24 = Colour	
	25 = Breeze	
	26 = Thought	

Question 1

Examine the following coded message:
(A, ҉), (A, 2), (6, 3)

Now examine the following sentences and try to determine the most likely interpretation of the code.

A The building made people happy

B I felt sad so I scampered home

C Happy people scampered towards the building

D I feel sad inside the building

E People in the building were happy

Question 2

Examine the following coded message:
(13, H, 1,) (15, H), 10

Now examine the following sentences and try to determine the most likely interpretation of the code.

A The sun reflected itself into the water

B The sun merged the ice into water

C The sun melted the ice, and the footprints melted into the sea

D The footprints, merged into the sea and the sun merged into the ice

E The sun melted the snow, and the footprints dissolved into the sea

Question 3

Examine the following coded message:
($\nearrow$, 2), (A, B), 6, 8

Now examine the following sentences and try to determine the most likely interpretation of the code.

A Daring people have a decreased risk of danger

B Daring people are dangerous runners

C Courageous people are more likely to run into danger

D Daring people are increasingly dangerous

E Daring is increasingly dangerous

Question 4

Examine the following coded message: (2, ♋), 3

Now examine the following sentences and try to determine which **two** are the most likely interpretations of the code.

A The church is held in a public trust

B People are trusting of strong buildings

C People trust their banks

D People are trusting

E Most buildings are sponsored by a public trust

Question 5

Examine the following coded message: (2,●), (A, B), 26

Now examine the following sentences and try to determine the most likely interpretation of the code.

A   Geniuses have a decreased anatomy

B   People who are intelligent have limited anatomy

C   Genius's brains are bigger in size

D   Intelligent anatomies greatly belong to humans

E   Humans are intelligent as they have larger anatomies

Question 6

Examine the following coded message:
(A, 19), I, 6, (20, 3), ❑

Now examine the following sentences and try to determine the most likely interpretation of the code.

A   She came running down the stairs, aggressively

B   He came running up the structure angry

C   He came running down the structure of the building

D   She ran up the stairs in a rage

E   She ran down the stairs angrily

Question 7

Examine the following coded message:
(21, 2), (A, J), (A, 8), 2

Now examine the following sentences and try to determine the most likely interpretation of the code.

A The security is strong and helps the public from danger

B The security keeps people safe

C The police are strong safe-guards of the public

D The police are professional members to keep the public safe

E The security keeps the structure safe

Question 8

Examine the following coded message: 5, 7, 11, 10

Now examine the following sentences and try to determine the most likely interpretation of the code.

A Yesterday it rained, tomorrow will be sandier

B Yesterday it rained, tomorrow will be dryer

C Yesterday the sand was wet

D Tomorrow the water will have sand inside it

E Yesterday and tomorrow the water will have sand

Question 9

Examine the following coded message:
4, (A, B), (A, D), 1, 10, 7

Now examine the following sentences and try to determine which **two** options are the most likely interpretations of the code.

A The sun shines over the city across the sand and sea

B The sun always shines in the city which never sleeps

C Cities usually have a lot of sunshine with many beaches

D Hot cities usually have sun and sand and very little water

E Cairo is very hot with sun, sea and sand

Question 10

Examine the following coded message:
22, 2, (A, ⌘, C), 8

Now examine the following sentences and try to determine the most likely interpretation of the code.

A People will always be in danger during natural disasters

B Natural dangers are always a liability for the public

C People are never calm during an earthquake

D People must remain calm during a natural disaster

E Natural disasters are very dangerous

Question 11

Examine the following coded message:
(2, A), (A, ◑, C), (◑), 2

Now examine the following sentences and try to determine the most likely interpretation of the code.

A I am a sociable person but I dislike other negative extraverts

B I am a very sociable person and I enjoy meeting people, but I dislike those who are shy and reserved

C I am an extravert and I enjoy meeting extraverted people

D I enjoy socialising

E I enjoy partying, however I dislike extraverted people

Question 12

Examine the following coded message: 4, 10, 1, (22, 8)

Now examine the following sentences and try to determine the most likely interpretation of the code.

A Natural disasters affect all countries

B Floods and droughts are a cause of natural disasters

C The city was flooded with rain

D The natural disasters struck the city, with water and sun

E The rain in London caused a flood but it soon dried up

Question 13

Examine the following coded message: 2, (13, 3), D

Now examine the following sentences and try to determine the 2 most likely interpretations of the code.

A   The snow falls on the roof tops

B   The residents of the Antarctic make their homes out of snow

C   The Inuit people live in cold igloos

D   Ice can be made in the freezer

E   Homes are always cold in the winter

Question 14

Examine the following coded message:
(24, 1), 2, 9, ⊬

Now examine the following sentences and try to determine the most likely interpretation of the code.

A   The shepherd's face was as red as the sun

B   The sun shone in the red sky, as the shepherds watched with delight

C   The sun will shine tonight

D   Happy people will be out tonight

E   Red sky at night, shepherds' delight

Question 15

Examine the following coded message: (17, A), H, 4, (A, 1)

Now examine the following sentences and try to determine the most likely interpretation of the code.

A The moonlight shone onto the darkness of the city

B The moon merged shyly into the darkness of the city

C The sun lit up the dark city

D The city lights lit up like the sun

E Lights in Las Vegas are as bright as the moon

Question 16

Examine the following coded message: 20, ⌘, 3

Now examine the following sentences and try to determine the most likely interpretation of the code.

A The building had a messy structure

B The composition of the building was in a terrible state

C The structure of the building was enormously unbalanced

D The walls of the house were crumbling

E The spiral staircase was very much unbalanced

Question 17

Examine the following coded message: 22, 8, (G, 7)

Now examine the following sentences and try to determine the most likely interpretation of the code.

A There is danger ahead as there is quicksand in the jungle

B The jungle is a very dangerous place as there are deep sandpits

C Quickly go into the jungle and run from danger

D Quicksand dangerously overflows the natural habitat

E Quicksand is one of nature's natural disasters

Question 18

Examine the following coded message: (A, J, 18), 2, ♓

Now examine the following sentences and try to determine the most likely interpretation of the code.

A Happy people have healthy bodies

B Happy people are strong

C Weak people are never happy with their bodies

D I am happy because my body is healthy

E Strong people have happy bodies

Question 19

Examine the following coded message:
(A, 2), (◆, ⌘), 2, (C, ♋)

Now examine the following sentences and try to determine the most likely interpretation of the code.

A   I do not trust shy people

B   Shy and unstable people should never be trusted

C   I feel inhibited and unsteady, that's why I do not trust other people

D   I am opposite to shy people

E   You can trust shy people but never the opposite

Question 20

Examine the following sentence *'He was hot headed as she was not trustworthy'*

Now examine the following codes and try to determine the most likely interpretation of the sentence.

A   □, 2, (C, □)

B   (C, □), 19, □

C   19, (A, 19), (C, ♋), □

D   19, □, (A, 19), (C, □)

E   19, (A, 19), □

THIS IS THE HALFWAY STAGE. IDEALLY YOU SHOULD HAVE APPROXIMATELY THIRTEEN MINUTES LEFT

(Please note this prompt will not be given in your actual test)

Question 21

Examine the following sentence: *'The strong hurricane made the structure of the buildings dangerous'*.

Now examine the following codes and try to determine the most likely interpretation of the sentence.

A   (J), 25, 8, 20

B   8, (22, 8, 25), 3, 20 (A, J)

C   (A, J), 25, 8, 20

D   (22, 8), 8, 4, 20, 3

E   25, J, 20, 3, 8

Question 22

Examine the following sentence: *'I find it easy to get on with self-assured people as I am gregarious myself'*.

Now examine the following codes and try to determine the most likely interpretation of the sentence.

A   A, K, ◯, 2, A, 2

B   ◯, 2, (A, 2)

C   (A, K), ◯, 2, (A, 2), ◯

D   (A, 2), 2, (K, 2), ◯

E   (A, 2), 2, K

Question 23

Examine the following sentence: *'People tend to float on the moon'*.

Now examine the following codes and try to determine the most likely interpretation of the sentence.

A A, 1, (A, 2)

B (A, 1), 2, 25

C A, 2, 25, 1

D (A, 1), 2, 25, 15

E (A, 1), 2

Question 24

Examine the following sentence: *'I dislike fire as it will burn me'*.

Now examine the following codes and try to determine the most likely interpretation of the sentence.

A A, 2, A, D, C, L

B 24, (A, 2), (A, D), (C, L)

C 2, (A, D), (C, L)

D (A, 2), (A, D), (C, L)

E (A, 2), (A, D), L

Question 25

Examine the following sentence: *'I dislike my light coloured eyes'*.

Now examine the following codes and try to determine the most likely interpretation of the sentence.

A 17, 18, (A, 2), 24, L

B (C, L), 2, 24, 18, 17

C C, L, 17, 18, A, 2, 24

D (C, L), 17, 18, (A, 2), 24, 7

E (C, L), 17, 18, (A, 2), 24

Question 26

Examine the following sentence: *'Audacious people prefer change rather than structure and stability'*.

Now examine the following codes and try to determine the most likely interpretation of the sentence.

A 2, (C, L), 20, L, (A, ⌘) ⌘, ↗

B 2, C, L, 20, L, A, ⌘, ⌘, ↗

C L, A, ⌘, ⌘, ↗,(C, L), 20

D (A, 2), (C, L), 20, L, (A, ⌘) ⌘, ↗

E 8, 2, (C, L), 20, L, (A, ⌘) ⌘, ↗

Verbal Reasoning answers and justifications

Question 1

> *It has been suggested that listening to music may develop an individual's imaginative ability. It can help people concentrate on thoughts, brainstorm ideas, help creativity in the formation of art and inventions and help people formulate solutions to complex tasks and theories. There have been examples of scientists who have exploited music to help them learn, give inspiration to introduce novel concepts and knowledge, and find solutions to complicated scientific notions. For example, Albert Einstein would often listen to a violin piece while deep in thought, trying to solve physics problems.*

A Listening to music will enhance a scientist's creativity

Answer: False

In the passage it is stated that listening to music 'may' enhance an individual's creativity, therefore there is not a definitive statement. However, the above statement makes a claim that it 'will' enhance creativity.

B *If an individual listened to classical music, originality may be achieved*

Answer: Can't tell

In the passage it is stated that listening to music may enhance ones creativity, however it is not stated which specific type of music may enhance creativity, and therefore the information is too limited to make a claim that classical music will develop imaginative ability.

C *Einstein developed solutions to various problems by playing a violin*

Answer: False

In the passage, it is noted that Einstein 'listened' to a violin rather than played one, therefore the statement is false based on the information given.

D *Listening to music will allow an individual to become more creative*

Answer: False

As mentioned previously, the passage states that there is a 'possibility' that listening to music will enhance an individual's creativity; the passage does not state this definitively.

Question 2

> Copper is usually used for the voice coil, however other metallic elements such as aluminium can also be utilised. The voice coil wire can be circular, rectangular or even hexagonal. A range of various voice coil wires are used in order to give different volume coverage, within a magnetic gap. The voice coil is positioned coaxially inside the gap. This gap is in actual fact a small circular hole, within the magnetic structure in order for the voice coil to be able to move back and fourth. This gap creates a powerful magnetic field amid the poles of a permanent magnet, whereby the outside of the gap acts as a singular pole, and the centre post serves as the other. The centre post and the back plate are known as the 'Yoke'.

A   Voice coil wires come in various geometrical shapes, such as circular in a two dimensional figure with five sides and five equal angles, or they can be a four sided plane figure with four right angles

Answer: False

The passage states that the voice coil can be circular, rectangular or even hexagonal. However in the statement it refers to a five sided shape i.e. a pentagon which is not mentioned in the passage. This means that the statement is false.

B *The small circular hole creates a robust magnetic field outside the poles of a magnet*

Answer: False

The fifth sentence states that the small circular hole creates a magnetic field 'inside' the poles of the magnet. In contrast to this, the above statement claims that the hole is outside the poles of the magnet.

C *A pole is situated at the hub of the magnetic field this is also known as the 'Yoke'*

Answer: False

Towards the end of the passage it is stated that the yoke combines the poles inside the centre of the magnetic field and the poles outside of the magnetic field, therefore the above statement is false.

D *There is a physical magnet in the voice coil*

Answer: True

Towards the end of the passage it is stated that there is a "magnetic field amid the poles of a permanent magnet". This means that a physical magnet does in fact exist.

Question 3

> *From October 2006, The Employment Equality (age) Regulations make it illegal to discriminate against workers, employers, jobseekers and trainees due to their age. Direct discrimination is set out in the regulations, and states that it is unlawful, on the grounds of age, to come to a decision about employing someone or dismissing someone, refuse to provide training, deny individuals promotion and make individuals work in adverse conditions.*
>
> *The second form of discrimination (indirect discrimination) is related to selection criteria, benefits, policies, and various employment rules and practises which may disadvantage particular people of specific ages, unless the practise which is utilised is justified.*
>
> *The regulation also allows organisations to predetermine the retirement age. This therefore means that one is able to set retirement ages at or above 65.*

A   A job vacancy specifically advertising for graduates is a form of discrimination

Answer: False

At first it may seem that the above statement is discriminative, however in reality it does not discriminate at all. Instead all the advertisement asks for are graduates, who can be of any age. Therefore it does not discriminate on the grounds of age.

B *Indirect discrimination refers only to an organisation's guiding principals*

Answer: False

The passage states that indirect discrimination relates to selection criteria; however an organisation's guiding principals are more related with direct discrimination, such as denying individuals promotion and making individuals work in adverse conditions.

C *The act will allow a 75 year old to be in employment*

Answer: True

Towards the end of the passage it is stated that an organisation is allowed to predetermine the retirement age, therefore this can be set at 65 years or over.

D *An organisation justifies that an 18 year old is unable to be considered as a candidate as he or she does not have the right qualifications. This is a form of age discrimination.*

Answer: False

The organisation has not selected the candidate based on their qualifications rather than their age. Therefore the above statement is incorrect.

Question 4

> *Applications are now being accepted for the following courses; advanced and foundation Danish, intermediate Ukrainian, advanced, intermediate and foundation Bulgarian, and finally intermediate and foundation Russian. All of the courses will include an Introductory Workshop, with the exception of the non-European languages. You can pick up an application form from the Institute of Foreign Arts; applications will need to be submitted by 10th March 2007. A 10% deposit will need to be paid in advance before the commencement of the course and thereafter payments can be made in four quarterly instalments at the end of each quarter. By the fourth instalment the course will be completed.*

A The institution only teaches European languages

   Answer: False

It is stated in the passage that there will be no introductory workshops for the non-European languages, therefore this reveals that the institute also teaches other languages. This means that the above statement is false.

B The course lasts for a whole year

   Answer: True

Towards the end of the passage it is stated that the course will need to be paid for in quarterly instalments. By the fourth instalment, the course will be completed. Four quarterly instalments consist of a total of twelve months; therefore it is true that the course lasts for a whole year.

C *The languages which the institute advertises courses for are all European*

Answer: True

The course only advertises information for the European languages, no further information is given about the non-European languages, and therefore the above statement is true.

D *The Institute of Foreign Arts has all the application forms*

Answer: Can't tell

The passage only states that the application forms for the language courses are available at the Institute of Foreign Arts; no further information is given as to whether the Institute has all the application forms.

Question 5

Although autism was first discovered in 1943, it is still a relatively unknown disability. Children with autism do not show any signs of physical disability. It is a lifelong development disability that affects an individual's social interaction, social imagination and communication skills. Most sufferers can often have learning difficulties.

A form of autism is called Asperger's syndrome, which is used to describe sufferers who are usually at the higher functioning end of the autistic spectrum. It seems that to an autistic person reality is a confusing, interacting mass of events, people, places, sounds, and sights. A sufferer may not have clear boundaries, order or meaning to anything.

A People who see an autistic child may assume they look 'normal'

Answer: True

At the beginning of the passage, it explains that autistic children do not show any signs of any physical disabilities, therefore we are able to make a claim that they look 'normal'.

B Autistic children may not have the ability to develop reciprocal relationships

Answer: True

The passage states that autistic children have difficulties with social interaction and this is a form of reciprocal relationship. Therefore the above statement is true.

C Autistic children are unable to make sense of their world

Answer: True

Towards the end of the passage, there is a section which describes that reality to an autistic child is confusing, and has no clear boundaries, order or meaning to anything. From this we can make a general inference that an autistic child is unclear about the world around them.

D Autistic children are able to comprehend and put forward new ideas about creative play

Answer: False

The passage states that autistic children have difficulties in terms of social imagination; therefore they have a difficulty in developing creative play. This therefore contradicts the above passage.

Question 6

The legislative maternity privileges shape a minimum standard of protection recognised by Parliament. Women and their employers (or their legislative bodies) are able to negotiate and consent to more constructive provision on a voluntary or contractual foundation, if they feel that this would be more beneficial in the long term. Where an employer and employee have agreed diverse provisions, an employee will always be able to declare her statutory rights if these are better than those agreed with her employer, therefore if the employee wishes a term by maternity privileges she is able to do so. This therefore means that an employee will not be obliged to accept maternity arrangements which are not as good as the legislative rights.

In order to qualify for Statutory Maternity Pay, an employee will have to be an employed earner, therefore the employee will need to work for an organisation that is liable to pay the employees share of National Insurance contributions.

To qualify for Maternity Allowance an employee must be, or have recently been either an employed or self-employed earner. The majority of people, who qualify for leave will also qualify for pay, and vice versa. All employees who are parents to new babies have a right to statutory leave with pay. However, there are a few legal clauses. For instance, the privileges relating to time off for antenatal care, to maternity leave and to protection against detriment or unfair dismissal in connection with maternity leave do not apply to the following groups: members of the police force,

> MPs, the judiciary and various company directors,
> or to masters or crew members engaged in share
> fishing paid solely by how much stock they have
> caught.

*A Women are entitled to all legislative maternity
privileges*

Answer: False

The above statement refers to all women being entitled
to legislative maternity privileges, however at the end of
the passage it is stated that there are certain limitations
on who is able to qualify for maternity allowance
such as members of the police force, MPs and so on.
Therefore the above statement is false as not all women
are entitled to these privileges.

*B In order for an individual to qualify for maternity
allowance, an employee will have to work for an
organisation who are liable to pay the employees'
share of National Insurance contributions*

Answer: False

The statement is false as it refers to 'Maternity Allowance'
instead of 'Statutory Maternity Pay' (where the grounds
to qualify are dependant on the employer paying the
employee's share of National Insurance contributions).
Do not make the mistake of assuming different terms
mean the same thing.

C *Men are allowed time off if they are a parent to a new baby*

Answer: True

The statement proposes that all parents to new babies are allowed time off work. Therefore the phrase 'All employees who are parents to new babies have a right for statutory leave with pay' refers to both men and women.

D *The rights described in the passage above only relate to employees and not those who are unemployed.*

Answer: True

The passage only relates to those who are in employment, there is no reference to those who are unemployed.

Question 7

Healthcare workers are at an increased risk of both fatal and non fatal injuries, due to a number of various factors ranging from violence within the workplace to apparatus being placed carelessly such as syringes and needles. However, recent research has found that there has been a decrease in medical and mental healthcare, and instead there is a high increase in the use of hospitals for severely disturbed violent cases, severe mental illness, drug abuse, or other types of out-of-the-ordinary behaviours by some patients. This form of violence is increasing in severity and frequency, in areas such as pharmacies, hospitals and community care facilities, and has now become a seemingly never-ending problem.

> It has been proposed that a resolution to such a problem would be to restrict the premature discharge of the chronically mentally ill from professional care services.

A   **Increased risk of injury to healthcare workers is wholly due to an increase in healthcare and a decrease in the hospitalisation of those with mental health problems**

   Answer: False

The passage states "There is now a decrease in medical and mental healthcare and instead there is a high increase in the use of hospitals for severely disturbed violent cases", therefore the statement is false.

B   **If hospitalised patients remain in specialist care for longer periods, a decrease in injuries may be seen**

   Answer: Can't tell

In the passage it is stated that healthcare workers are at risk due to various factors, ranging from violence to carelessly placed apparatus. It has been proposed that if mentally ill patients stayed in hospital longer, there may be a reduction in violent cases. However, there is no further information given to see the effects of this proposed solution, hence we are unable to conclude whether the proposal had any beneficial effects.

C *Individuals who show atypical behaviours have been shown to be hospitalised*

Answer: True

The second sentence states that individuals who have shown out of the ordinary behaviours have been known to be hospitalised.

D *All mentally ill patients show violent behaviours*

Answer: False

In the passage it is suggested that *some* mentally ill patients show violent behaviours. In contrast, the above statement generalises that all mentally ill patients show violent behaviours. This therefore makes the above statement false, based on the information given in the passage.

Question 8

Marketing and advertising books via various internet sites is becoming most popular with traders. This is chiefly because it costs less to publicise the actual book, as compared to traditional methods such as conferences and advertisements on billboards and in newspapers. Books are also stored in large warehouses prior to being dispatched to customers, nationally and internationally. Therefore overheads are also less. Whilst this may be true, publishers feel that they are not gaining an adequate amount from book sales, and are not just demanding that they are paid for the cover prices of the books, but also that they receive a percentage of the actual amount received for them. However, these discounts only seem possible on books which are bestsellers.

A *The consumer demand for books which are sold over the internet is increasing*

   Answer: Can't tell

The information in the passage only states how popular the internet is becoming for marketing purposes, however there is no further information given to make conclusions about consumer demand.

B *The general recurring costs of running a publishing business are high*

   Answer: False

In the passage it is stated that the overheads or overall costs of running the business are less, in contrast to the above statement which states that the overheads are high.

C *Internet bookstores tender the greatest concession on the least popular books*

   Answer: Can't tell

The passage does not state that *general* discounts are given on the least popular books, instead it only mentions discounts given to publishers on their best sellers, therefore there is no further information available on which to base a decision.

D *Conventional methods of publicising a book are more expensive*

   Answer: True

The passage states that "It costs less to publicise the actual book, when compared to *traditional methods* such as conferences and advertisements on billboards and in newspapers", therefore the above statement is true, based on the information given in the passage.

Question 9

Cardiovascular Disease (CVD) cost the healthcare system around £14,750 million in 2003, which works out a cost per person of just below £250. 76% of these costs were towards hospital healthcare and 18% can be accounted for by drugs and dispensing.

Coronary Heart disease (CHD) cost the healthcare system around £3,500 million in 2003, which works out a cost per person of just below £60. 79% of these costs were put towards hospital care and 16% towards drugs and dispensing.

There are also non healthcare costs including those from 'Production losses' from death and illness in those who were in employment. Informal care of people with the disease greatly adds to the financial burden.

In 2003, CVD related production losses stood at £6,200 million due to mortality and morbidity, with approximately 60% of this cost specifically due to death and 40% due to illness in those of working age. The cost of informal care for people with CVD was just over £4,800 million in 2003.

In 2003, production losses due to mortality and morbidity associated with CHD cost over £3,100 million, with around 30% of this cost specifically due to death and 70% due to illness in those of working age, stalling by 10% when compared to previous costs in 2002. The cost of informal care for people with CHD was around £1,250 million in 2003.

A *The overall healthcare system costs for CHD and CVD increased by at least 49.1% when compared to the overall production losses*

Answer: True

This statement requires some simple addition. We first find the totals of the healthcare costs for CHD and CVD which was £18,250 million. We then find the overall production losses for CHD and CVD combined, which was £9,300 million. The next step is to find the difference between the two, which is equal to £8,950 million. We take this sum (£8,950) and divide it by the original total we are comparing against which is £18,250 million and multiply by 100, which gives a percentage of 49.1% (rounded to 1 decimal point).

B *The per capita cost for CVD was relatively higher than the per capita cost for CHD*

Answer: True

When we refer to per capita costs, we are really identifying the cost per person, therefore the per capita cost for CVD was £250 per person and £60 per person for those with CHD. Therefore this means that the above statement is true, as there is a difference of £190 between the per capita costs of CVD and CHD.

C *There are a total of approximately 59 million patients on whom the CVD costs are based*

Answer: True

This question again requires simple mental arithmetic: we first find out the total of the costs for each per capita, which for CVD is £14,750 million. From this we then divide the total costs by the costs per person. Therefore for CVD, the cost per person is £250. We then carry out the following calculation, which is total costs, divided by the costs per person: therefore for CVD the calculation will be £14,750 million divided by 250, which equals 59 million people.

D *The production losses specifically due to death for CHD are higher than those production losses related to CVD*

   Answer: (False)

In the passage, it is stated that the production losses due to death for CHD were 30% of £3,100 million, therefore we first need to determine 30% of £3,100 million. We do this by dividing £3,100 million by 100 and multiplying it by 30, which equals £930 million. We do the same calculation for CVD whereby the production losses due to death were 60% of £6200 million. Therefore we find that 60% of 6200 equals £3720 million.

Therefore the production losses due to death for CHD were in fact lower than production losses due to death for CVD. This means that the above statement is incorrect.

Question 10

The Scottish and Newcastle brewery have blamed the unpredictable weather for the drop in their profits for the year 2007. Statistics show last years net profits of £76 million had dropped by 9% in the first six months of this year compared to the same period the previous year. The wet weather has been prominent throughout summer and, due to the fact that there is no large sporting event such as the 2006 football World Cup to increase sales, this has led to a further 4.3% drop for the

> remainder of the year. The chairman of Scottish and Newcastle has claimed that the continuation of this bad weather in the UK and France will make it most challenging to reach this year's target.
>
> The Fosters beer company introduced a new low calorie line in 2006 with the intention of inflating their profits. This inflated Fosters' 2006 profits by 55.5%. This figure is still rising today. While the profits for Fosters low calorie beer continue to rise, the proportion of the original Fosters' profits were 50% of Scottish and Newcastle's previous net profits.

A   *Scottish and Newcastle's profits in 2007 were £65.9 million*

   Answer: True

It is stated in the passage that Scottish and Newcastle's, profits were a total of 13.3% (9% + 4.3%) less than their last year's profits of £76 million. We first need to find out what 13.3% of £76 million is. We do the following calculation: 13.3 divided by 100 multiplied by 76 million = 10.108. We then subtract this total from the original figure for 2006 which was £76 million (£76 million – £10.108 million = £65.9 million to 1 decimal place).

B   *The 'original' Fosters line profits for 2007 are £38 million*

   Answer: True

It is stated in the passage that the profit for the original Fosters line was 50% of Scottish and Newcastle's previous net profit, which was £76million. 50% of £76 million = £38 million.

C *The breweries are suffering profit decrease due to long periods of bad weather*

   Answer: Can't tell

No further information is given as to what is classified as long periods of weather, hence we are unable to conclude the above statement.

D *Fosters' profits from 2006 and 2007 are lower than the profits Scottish and Newcastle breweries made in 2006*

   Answer: Can't tell

We are not given any further information on the total of Fosters' profits for 2006 to 2007, as there is limited information given on the Fosters' low calorie drink. Hence we are unable to conclude the above statement.

Question 11

The Santa Monica is a well defined unit of transverse mountain ranges in Southern California, situated at the core of the island. These ranges are perpendicular to the coast of Sierra Nevada and the Pennsylvania ranges. A mile of pink blossom trees brightens the pathway of each peak. Santa Monica, or 'the high one' as it is known, is often hidden away in the heavens. On a winter's day, one can see only the barks of blossom trees. Each mountain top has a layer of snow like icing on a cake. The triple peaks glisten like diamonds in a river, beneath the sunshine over the heart of the coast. Opposite Santa Monica lies its twin, Santa Louisa with three snow-layered peaks. However, Santa Louisa still looks like a baby when compared to 'the high one'.

A *Mount Santa Monica is to be found at the heart of the island*

Answer: True

It is stated in the passage that the mountain ranges are found at the core of the island, or the centre of the island.

B *The Mountain has an identical twin across the island*

Answer: False

In the passage it is stated that the Santa Louisa is a twin of the Santa Monica, but the passage goes on to say that the Santa Louisa mountain range is still a 'baby', therefore we are able to infer that they are smaller and therefore not an identical twin to the Santa Monica mountain range.

C *Santa Monica is high enough to almost reach the sky*

Answer: True

It is stated in the passage that the mountain ranges are high enough to reach the heavens; therefore we can use heavens as a metaphor for the skies.

D *The Santa Monica is at right angles to the coast of Sierra Nevada*

Answer: True

It is stated in the passage that 'these ranges are perpendicular to the coast of Sierra Nevada and the Pennsylvania ranges'. Perpendicular is another word for being at right angles, so the above statement is true.

Quantitative Reasoning
answers and justifications

| Question 1 | **Answer D** |

Step 1 — We need to look under the heading which provides information regarding readership figures for males and females in 1998.

Step 2 — Then compare the difference between each book read between males and females.

13% of females and 10% of males read 'Alive in the Past'. Therefore this book has the greatest female readership.

| Question 2 | **Answer B** |

Step 1 — We need to combine the readership for all the books; therefore we add the total readership of the following books in 1981:

(Alive in the Past) 6.9 + (A Warm Day) 2.2 + (My Best Friend) 2.9 = 12 million readers

| Question 3 | **Answer A** |

Step 1 — Find the difference between the two readership figures:

6.9 million (1981) – 4.8 million (1998) = 2.1 million

| Step 2 | Find the percentage decrease, which is calculated by dividing the previous difference by the original number of readers (i.e. 6.9 million): |

2.1 ÷ 6.9 x 100 = 30.43%

Question 4   **Answer B**

| Step 1: | In 1998 it shows in the table that there are 8.9 million readers. |
| Step 2: | We know that a total of 22% of the adults surveyed read this book in 1998. |

We need to calculate how many males read the book so:

(8900000 ÷ 100) x 22 = 1958000 male readers

Question 5   **Answer A**

| Step 1 | We first determine how many boys had a low pulse rate. The table illustrates that out of 141 boys, 73 of them had a low pulse rate |
| Step 2 | We then need to determine what percentage 73 is of 141. We calculate this by dividing 73 by 141 and multiplying the total by 100: |

(73 ÷ 141) x 100 = 51.8%

Question 6   **Answer B**

Step 1   We first need to determine the total number of children who had a high pulse rate – this includes both boys and girls. There are a total of 129 children with high pulse rates.

Step 2   Secondly, we divide the total above by the total number of children who have both low and high pulse rates and multiply this by 100, to find the percentage:

(number of children with high pulse rates ÷ total number of children with both high and low pulse rates) x 100

129 ÷ 274 x 100 = 47.1%

Question 7   **Answer E**

Step 1   Using the formula in the above question we calculate the percentage in the following way:

(total number of girls in the group ÷ total number of children in the group) x 100

(133 ÷ 274) x 100= 48.5%

Question 8   **Answer E**

This question simply asks what the mode of all the childrens' pulse rates are, or in other words which score or group reoccurs the most:

61, 68, **73, 73**, 133,

= Girls' and boys' low pulse rate

Question 9 **Answer C**

The mean is worked out by adding the prices of all the items together and dividing by the number of items there are:

(3.20 + 1.20 + 1.00 + 2.00 +1.00 + 2.39) ÷ 6 = £1.7983 (1.80 to the nearest penny)

Question 10 **Answer C**

The median is a value which divides a sample of numbers into two equal parts.

In order to find out the median of the price list, we need to arrange all of the prices in ascending order and then find the middle value or pair. If there is a pair of values, we add the two values together and divide by two.

Step 1 3.20, 2.39, **2.00**, **1.20**, 1.00, 1.00

Step 2 **(£2.00 + £1.20) ÷ 2 = £1.60**

Question 11 **Answer C**

The range is found by subtracting the lowest item on the list from the highest item in the list.

£3.20 – £1.00 = £2.20

Question 12   **Answer D**

We need to add the totals of the range, the median and the mean, which have all been worked out in the previous questions within this section:

1.80 + 2.20 + 1.60 = £5.60

Question 13   **Answer E**

We need to find out the total number of graduates there are within the Teaching sector. The pie chart only shows percentages of the number of staff in each sector. No value is given, however we do know that the percentages are based on a total number of 166. The following formula calculates the values:

(Percentage ÷ 100) x total number of staff members in all sectors

(20 ÷ 100) x 166 = 33.2 (33 to the nearest whole number)

Question 14   **Answer B**

Step 1   We first find out how many people there are in the given sectors using the above formula:

Retail = (20 ÷ 100) x 166 = 33.2 (33 to the nearest whole number)

Freelance = (14 ÷ 100) x 166 = 23.24 (23 to the nearest whole number)

Step 2   Find the difference between the numbers of staff members in the two sectors:

33 − 23 = 10

There are 10 more staff members in Retail than in Freelance.

Question 15   Answer A

Step 1   To find out how many staff there are in each sector, we perform the following calculation:

(Percentage ÷ 100) x total number of staff members in all sectors

Finance = (13 ÷ 100) x 166 = 21.58 (22, to nearest whole number)

Business & Sales = (13 ÷ 100) x 166 = 21.58 (22, to nearest whole number)

Step 2   Add the total number of staff together:

22 + 22 = 44 members of staff are in Finance and Business & Sales

Question 16   Answer C

To answer this question we need to find the two figures and try to reduce them equally.

In the Teaching sector there are 33 members

In the Retail sector there are also 33 members.

Step 1   We can then say that the ratio of those in Teaching to those in Retail is 33:33.

Step 2   We can still reduce the above numbers further, by dividing them both equally, for example, if we divide both figures by 33, we can reduce the ratio to 1:1.

Therefore for every person in the Teaching sector there is an equal number in the Retail sector.

Question 17   **Answer E**

In the table we are given information about the total chain production, and standard chains on their own. However there is no information for how many substandard chains there are. This is for you to work out.

Step 1   In September the total chain production was 85 and the total standard production was 65. To find the substandard total, we subtract the total standard chains from the total chain production:

Substandard chain production = Total chain production – Standard chain production

85 – 65 = 20 substandard chains produced

Step 2   We then need to calculate this as a percentage of the total chain production:

(Total number of substandard chains ÷ total number of chain production) x 100

(20 ÷ 85) x 100 = 23.5%

Question 18   **Answer D**

Step 1   We first need to calculate how many standard and substandard chains there were in both October's and November's total sales value (see question 17):

October	Standard	-	80
	Substandard	-	20
November	Standard	-	85
	Substandard	-	10

Step 2   We then find out the cost of one standard chain and one substandard chain:

Standard chains cost £5.70 per 100
For one chain it is £5.70 ÷ 100 = £0.057 per standard chain.

Substandard chains cost £2.85 per 100
For one chain it is £2.85 ÷ 100 = £0.0285 per sub standard chain.

Step 3   We find the sales value of the standard and substandard chains for each month:

October	Standard	- 80 x 0.057
		= £4.56
	Substandard	- 20 x 0.0285
		= £0.57

November Standard   - 85 x 0.057
                              = £4.845
              Substandard - 10 x 0.0285
                              = £0.285

Step 4   We then add the total sales values of both months:

October   **£4.56 + £0.57= £5.13**

November   **£4.845 + £0.285= £5.13**

Question 19   **Answer E**

In October 20 substandard chains and 80 standard chains were produced, therefore we can write this as 20:80.

We can then reduce the above ratio by dividing each side by 20:

$20 \div 20 = 1$
$80 \div 20 = 4$

The ratio is now 1:4. Hence for every substandard chain produced there are 4 standard chains.

Question 20   **Answer E**

We take the substandard chains and divide them by the total chain production and multiply this figure by 100:

$(10 \div 70)$ x 100 = 14.29%

Question 21   **Answer B**

To determine this you add up all the totals from each group for each year and compare the differences.

Year 1 = 60 + 55 + 65 + 80 + 85 + 90 = 435 Sales staff

Year 2 = 70 + 60 + 85 + 100 + 95 + 100 = 510 Sales staff

Year 3 = 65 + 45 + 65 + 35 + 65 + 25 = 300 Sales staff

Question 22   **Answer B**

To determine this, add all the staff totals in each group for year 3:

Year 3 = 65 + 45 + 65 + 35 + 65 + 25 = 300

Question 23   **Answer E**

Step 1   You first need to find out how many staff members there were in years 1 and 3 in product group 4:

Year 1 = 80

Year 2 = 35

This means that there were 45 more staff members in year 1 than in year 3 (80 − 35 = 45).

Step 2   You then take the above difference and divide it by the number of staff in year 1 (to calculate percentage decrease). Then multiply it by 100 to achieve a percentage:

(45 ÷ 80) x 100 = 56.25 % (to 2 decimal places)

Question 24   **Answer C**

Step 1   Find the total number of staff members in year 1:

Year 1 = 60 + 55 + 65 + 80 + 85 + 90 = 435

Step 2   To find the mean, divide the above total by the number of product groups which is 6:

435 ÷ 6 = 72.5

Question 25   **Answer E**

The question asks how many garage doors are ≤ than 6.9 metres. The ≤ symbol means 'equal to or less than'.

Therefore there are 4 doors which are less than or equal to 5 – 5.9 metres and 12 doors which are less than or equal to 6 – 6.9 metres.

We then add the totals of these doors which gives us:

4 (5 – 5.9 metre doors) + 12 (6 – 6.9 metre doors) = 16

Question 26   **Answer D**

In total there are 32 out of 92 doors which have a height of less than 7.9 meters.

As a fraction this can be written as 32/92.

Step 1   We can still reduce this fraction to its
                simplest form by dividing it by 4:

                $32 \div 4 = 8$

                $92 \div 4 = 23$

                **The fraction can now be written as
                8/23**

Question 27   Answer C

                There are 12 doors in the range of 6
                – 6.9 metres and 24 in the range 8 -8.9
                metres. Hence the ratio is 12:24. As
                ratios are written in their lowest form,
                each number can be divided by 12 to
                achieve a ratio of:

                1:2

                Therefore there is 1 door of 6 – 6.9
                metres to every 2 doors of 8 – 8.9
                metres.

Question 28   Answer C

Step 1   We first need to know how many
                centimetres there are in 1 metre.

                In 1 metre there are 100cm.

                Therefore in 12.9 metres there are 1290
                cm (12.9 x 100).

Step 2   The question states that there are 5
                garage doors, therefore we need to
                multiply the above total by 5:

                1290 x 5 = 6450 cm

Question 29   **Answer C**

Step 1   You first need to calculate how much the maintenance contract would cost per year.

In the table it states that the maintenance contract costs £150.00 per month, therefore we need to multiply the monthly cost by 12 to find an annual payment:

150 x 12 = £1800.00

Step 2   We then need to find out how many call outs we need to make in a year for the contact to represent value for money. We do this by dividing the above sum by the call out charge not under a maintenance contract:

1800.00 ÷ 456.00 = 3.9 (4 call outs to the nearest whole number)

Question 30   **Answer B**

Step 1   We first determine the total cost of 12 call outs not under a maintenance contract:

12 x £456.00 = £5472.00

Step 2   The plumber then adds a 25% profit onto the above cost.

We then determine 25% of £5472.00 by calculating the following:

(25 ÷ 100) x 5472.00 = £1368.00 profit

Question 31   **Answer D**

Step 1   First find out the total cost of the maintenance contract for 1 year:

Monthly cost = £150.00

Yearly cost = 150 x 12= £1800

Step 2   We now multiply the above total by 3 as we are trying to find out the cost of the contract for 3 years:

£1800 x 3 = £5400.00

Step 3   Finally we need to work out a 12% discount on the total amount of the contract:

$(12 \div 100)$ x £5616.00 = £648.00

Step 4   We now subtract the 12% discount from the total cost of the maintenance contract for 3 years:

£5400.00 – £648.00 = £4752.00

Question 32   **Answer B**

Step 1   We first find out the following:

12 call outs not under a maintenance contract = £456 x 12 = £5472.00

4 call outs under a maintenance contract = £150 x 4 = £600.00

Step 2   We then take the totals of both the contracts and divide them by 30 to find out the daily rate the plumber got paid.

(£5472.00 + £600.00) $\div$ 30 = £202.40 per day

Question 33   **Answer B**

To calculate the number of Bulgarian Levs you can exchange for £45.00, you need to calculate the following:

£45.00 x 21 (BGL exchange rate) = 945 Levs

Question 34   **Answer D**

To calculate how much 677 Bangladeshi Takas are worth in Pounds Sterling you need to perform the opposite of the calculation in the above question:

677 ÷ 2.4 = £282.1 (1 decimal place)

Question 35   **Answer E**

Step 1   First find a 10% increase in the exchange rate for the Cuban Peso:

(10 ÷ 100) x 213 CUPs = 21.3

Step 2   Next we add the 10% increase to the original exchange rate:

21.3 + 213 = 234.3 *(New exchange rate for Cuban Peso)*

Step 3   Now we need to find out how many Cuban Pesos you would need to make £45.00:

£45.00 x 234.3 = 10543.5 CUPs

Question 36 **Answer C**

This question requires you to identify the actual exchange rate. We can work this out by the following calculation:

6790 ÷ 1900 = 3.6 (to 1 decimal place)

Question 37 **Answer C**

Step 1 We need to first identify how much chocolate you would need for one person. This can be calculated by dividing by 4 the amount of chocolate needed for 4 people:

256 ÷ 4 = 64g per person

Step 2 We then multiply the individual sum by 11 to find out the total amount of chocolate needed for 11 people:

64 x 11 = 704g of chocolate

Step 3 Chocolate is sold in 200g bars

3 blocks = 3 x 200 = 600g

4 blocks = 3 x 200 = 800g

We need 704g of chocolate so would therefore need to purchase 4 bars.

Question 38 **Answer E**

Step 1 Just like the previous question we need to find out how much margarine is needed per person:

124 ÷ 4 = 31g per person

Step 2	We then divide the amount of margarine in the recipe by 31 to determine how many people the recipe is based on:

1705 ÷ 31 = 55 people

Question 39	**Answer A**

Step one	We first need to find out the total amount of ingredients:

689 (grams of flour) + 100 (grams of sugar) + 124 (grams of margarine) + 256 (grams of chocolate) = 1169 grams of ingredients

Step 2	100 grams of sugar, expressed as a percentage of 1169 grams of total ingredients is:

(100 ÷ 1169) x 100 = 8.55% to 2 decimal places.

Question 40	**Answer D**

There are 124 grams of margarine to 256 grams of chocolate present in the recipe. This can be written as 124:256

However, this can be reduced further by dividing both numbers by 4:

124 ÷ 4 = 31

256 ÷ 4 = 64

31:64 (31 grams of margarine is required for every 64 grams of chocolate)

Abstract Reasoning
answers and justifications

Question 1

Set A

In this set there are black circles, white circles, a large star and an arrow present in each of the six boxes. The rules in this set are as follows:

1. There are always two black circles present in each test shape.

2. One white star is always present at a random position, but never towards a corner of the test shape.

3. One arrow is present facing north and is always placed towards the left hand side of the test shape.

4. The white circles are used as distracters.

Set B

In this set there are black circles, white circles, a large star and an arrow present in each of the six boxes. The rules in this set are as follows:

1. The star is always positioned at one of the corners of the test shape.

2. The arrows all face west and are positioned either at the top of the test shape or towards the bottom.

3. The black and white circles are used as distracters.

Test Shape 1 – Neither

The test shape incorporates rules of both sets. It appears to be related to Set A, as the test shape contains an arrow facing north which is positioned at the far left of the test shape. There are also two black circles present. However, the star is positioned towards the corner of the test shape which follows the rules of Set B, and ignores the rule of Set A whereby the star shape should be positioned anywhere in the test shape apart from by one of the corners.

Test Shape 2 – Set A

There are two black circles and an arrow facing north which is positioned towards the left hand side of the test shape. There is also a star shape present which is positioned almost towards the centre of the test shape. This therefore indicates that this test shape applies the rules of Set A. The test shape cannot belong to Set B for two reasons. The star shape is not positioned towards one of the corners of the test shape, and the arrow is not facing west and is not positioned at the top or bottom of the test shape.

Test Shape 3 – Set B

The test shape incorporates the rules of Set B, as the star shape is positioned in the bottom right hand corner of the test shape. Together with this, the arrow is facing west and is positioned at the bottom of the test shape. There is a black circle and a white circle present but these shapes are used as distracters. The test shape cannot be related to Set A as the star shape is positioned at the corner of the test shape, the arrow does not face north and is not positioned towards the left hand side of the test shape. Finally, there is only one black circle present instead of two.

Test shape 4 – Neither

The shape is not related to either set as the arrow is positioned at the corner of the test shape, and faces north-east. The test shape ignores the rules of both sets, whereby the arrow in Set A should face north and be positioned towards the left hand side of the test shape. Conversely, the arrow in Set B should be positioned either at the top or bottom of the test shape and face west.

Test Shape 5 – Neither

At first the test shape looks similar to Set A as there are two black circles, one star which is positioned in the centre of the test shape and an arrow positioned towards the left hand side of the test shape and facing north. However, upon closer inspection the arrow is in fact shorter than the arrows which are present in Set A.

Question 2

Set A

In this set there are large symmetrical shapes made from straight lines only. The main rule in this set is that, for each shape, there must be at least one or more triangular shapes, either within or outside of shapes. The white circles are used as distracters.

Set B

In this set there are large symmetrical shapes which are made from straight lines only. In this set the circles are in pairs or threes and the triangles are used as distracters.

Test Shape 1 – Set B

The test shape belongs to Set B, as the circles are presented in a pair. As well as this, the large shape is symmetrical and made of straight lines. The test shape cannot belong to Set A, as there are no corresponding triangles.

Test Shape 2 – Set B

The explanation for this test shape is identical to that for the test shape 1.

Test Shape 3 – Neither

The test shape does not belong to either group as the large shape is curved. Both sets have the characteristic of having one large shape which is made up of straight lines only.

Test Shape 4 – Neither

The large shape is not symmetrical, which is a requirement of both sets.

Test Shape 5 – Set A

There are three triangles, and a triangle present is a requirement of Set A. The test shape cannot belong to Set B as there is only one circle instead of two or three.

Question 3

Set A

There are various large symmetrical shapes present, consisting of a star, a rounded rectangle, an arrow, an oval, a smiley face and a cross with arrows on the edges. There are also small white and black stars present.

The rules in this set are as follows:

1. The large symmetrical shape should be made from dotted lines.

2. The black and white stars are used as distracters.

Set B

There are various symmetrical shapes present, including a rectangle blended with an arrow facing north, a cross, another arrow, a triangle, a rectangle and a 24 pointed star.

The rules in this set are as follows:

1. The symmetrical shape should comprise of solid lines.

2. The dotted lines and the shaded shapes present within the symmetrical shapes are used as distracters.

Test Shape 1 – Set A

The heart shape is symmetrical and comprises of a dotted outline. This test shape cannot belong in Set B as the outline must be solid.

Test Shape 2 – Neither

The outline of the shape is dotted so the test shape does seem similar to Set A. However, the shape is not symmetrical and therefore does not belong to either set.

Test Shape 3 – Set B

The shape is symmetrical and comprises a solid outline as per the rule of Set B. The inside of the shape contains a small circle with a dotted outline; however this test shape cannot belong to Set A, as the outline of the large shape is not dotted.

Test Shape 4 – Neither

The test shape does have a dotted outline, suggesting that it might belong to Set A. However, the shape is not symmetrical and therefore does not belong to either set.

Test Shape 5 – Set A

The large symmetrical shape has a dotted outline and black and white star shapes are present as distracters, therefore following the rules of Set A. The test shape cannot belong to Set B as the large shape does not have a solid outline.

Question 4

Set A

There are various large shapes present, consisting of a triangle, a rectangle, a square, a cross, an arrow and a diamond. There are also randomly placed smaller shapes consisting of a rectangle and a diamond.

1. There is only one consistent rule within this set which is that all of the shapes must contain at least one right angle.

Set B

There are various large shapes, consisting of a boat shape, a star, a heart, a curved rectangle, a circle and a lightning bolt. Two small squashed stars are placed in two of the boxes.

1. Again there is only one rule; the shapes should not comprise any right angles.

Test Shape 1 – Set A

Both shapes contain a right angle so the test shape therefore follows the rules of Set A

Test Shape 2 – Neither

Neither set comprises a combination of one shape containing right angles and one shape that does not, therefore this test shape does not follow the rules of either set.

Test Shape 3 – Set B

The shapes contain no right angles and therefore this test shape follows the rules of Set B.

Test Shape 4 – Set B

The test shape contains no right angles so therefore follows the rules of Set B.

Test Shape 5 – Set A

The test shape contains right angles and therefore follows the rules of Set A.

Question 5

Set A

In this set there are small triangular, rectangular and diamond/square shapes present.

The rules in this set are as follows:

1. When there are three rectangular shapes present there should be two triangular shapes present.

2. When there are four triangular shapes present there should be one rectangular shape present.

3. The diamond/square shapes are used as distracters.

Set B

In this set there are small triangular, rectangular and diamond shapes present.

The rules in this set are as follows:

1. When there are four rectangular shapes present there should be one diamond/square shape present.

2. When there are four diamond/square shapes present there should be one rectangular shape present.

3. The triangular shapes are used as distracters.

Test Shape 1 – Set B

There are four rectangular shapes and one diamond shape present, which means that this test shape follows the rules of Set B. The test shape does not follow the rules of Set A, as the pattern of three rectangles to one triangle is not present.

Test shape 2 – Set A

There are four triangular shapes and one rectangular shapes present. Therefore the test shape follows the rules of Set A. The test shape does not follow the rules of Set B as there are only three diamond/squares present instead of one or four.

Test Shape 3 – Neither

The test shape contains no rectangular shapes, and therefore does not follow the rules of either set.

Test Shape 4 – Set A

There are four triangular shapes for every rectangular shape present. This shape does not follow the rules of Set B as there are only three diamond/square shapes present instead of one or four.

Test Shape 5 – Neither

There are five triangular shapes present instead of two or four, hence the test shape does not follow the rules of Set A. The test shape does not follow the rules of Set B either as there are no diamond/square shapes present.

Question 6

Set A

In this set there should only be three circular/oval shapes, which are of different sizes; small, medium and large. The smallest shape should always be within the largest shape.

Set B

In a similar way to Set A, there should only be three circular/oval shapes present, which are of different sizes; small, medium and large. Set B differs from Set A in that the smallest shape should be placed within the medium sized shape.

Test Shape 1 – Set B

The test shape belongs to Set B, as the smallest shape is within the medium sized shape. The test shape cannot belong to Set A, as the smallest shape would need to be within the largest shape.

Test Shape 2 – Set A

The test shape belongs to Set A, as the smallest shape is within the largest shape. The test shape cannot belong to Set B, as the smallest shape would need to be within the medium sized shape.

Test Shape 3 – Neither

The smallest circular shape is not within the large or medium sized shape, therefore it does not follow the rules of either set.

Test Shape 4 – Neither

As above, the smallest shape is not within any shape, and again does not follow the rules of either set.

Test Shape 5 – Set A

The test shape belongs to Set A, as the smallest shape is within the largest shape. The test shape cannot belong to Set B, as the smallest shape would need to be within the medium sized shape.

Question 7

Set A

There are various large symmetrical shapes present, which comprise of dashed outlines. There are smaller shapes present within these large shapes which have a solid outline and are either filled black or filled white.

Rules:

1. The test shape must be symmetrical.
2. The test shape must comprise of a dashed outer line.
3. The distracters are the black and white small shapes, which have a solid outer line.

Set B

There are various large symmetrical shapes present, which have a solid outline. There are smaller shapes within these large shapes which have both solid and dashed outlines and are either filled black or filled white.

Rules:

1. The test shape must be symmetrical.

2. The test shape must have a solid outline.

3. The distracters are the black and white filled small shapes, which have either a solid or dashed outline.

Test Shape 1 – Set A

The test shape is symmetrical and has a dashed outline, therefore follows the rules of Set A. This test shape cannot be part of Set B, as it does not have a solid outline.

Test Shape 2 – Set B

The test shape is symmetrical and has a solid outline. This test shape cannot be part of Set A as it does not have a dashed outline.

Test Shape 3 – Neither

The test shape comprises a dashed outline and seems similar to Set A. However, the shape is not symmetrical and therefore cannot be related to either set.

Test Shape 4 – Neither

The test shape has a solid outline and first appears to follow the rules of Set B. However, as in the previous question, the test shape is not symmetrical and therefore cannot be related to either set.

Test Shape 5 – Set B

The test shape is symmetrical and has a solid outline, and therefore follows the rules of Set B. This shape cannot belong to Set A as it does not have a dashed outline.

Question 8

Set A

In this set there are a variety of large symmetrical shapes which have a curved or straight dashed outline. There are also smaller curved shapes which have a solid outline positioned within or outside of the larger shapes.

Set B

In this set there are a variety of large symmetrical shapes which have a straight or curved dashed outline. Each shape must have a rectangle, whether within shapes or outside shapes.

Test Shape 1 – Set B

The test shape belongs to Set B, as there is a small rectangle alongside the large heart shape. The test shape does not belong to Set A, as the smaller shape is not curved.

Test Shape 2 – Set B

The test shape belongs to Set B, as there are two small rectangles alongside the large triangle shape. The test shape does not belong to Set A, as the smaller shape is not curved.

Test Shape 3 – Neither

The shape cannot belong to either set as it does not have a dashed outline.

Test Shape 4 – Set A

The test shape belongs to Set A as there are two circles within each other. The outer circle has a dashed outline while the circle inside has a solid outline. The test shape does not belong to Set B as there are no rectangles present.

Test Shape 5 – Neither

The test shape looks closer to Set B as there are rectangles within the parallelogram. However, it is not symmetrical and therefore cannot belong to this set.

Question 9

Set A

The set contains small rectangular, circular and crescent shapes.

The rules followed are:

1. Where there are four circular shapes present, there should be two rectangular shapes present.

2. Where there are four rectangular shapes present, there should be two circular shapes present.

3. The crescent shapes are used as distracters.

Set B

The set contains small rectangular, circular and crescent shapes.

The rules are as follows:

1. Where there are four circular shapes present, there should be two crescent shapes present.

2. Where there are four crescent shapes present, there should be two circular shapes present.

3. The rectangular shapes are used as distracters.

Test Shape 1 – Set A

There are four rectangular shapes present together with two circular shapes which follows the pattern of Set A. This test shape cannot belong to Set B as when two circular shapes are present there should be four crescent shapes present, but in this test shape there are actually five.

Test Shape 2 – Neither

The test shape comprises five rectangular shapes and therefore cannot be part of Set A, which requires that four rectangular shapes are present to every two circular shapes. The test shape cannot be related to Set B as there are not two circular shapes to four crescent shapes present.

Test Shape 3 – Neither

The test shape comprises three rectangular shapes and four circular shapes and therefore is not related to Set A, as there must be four rectangular shapes to two circular shapes. The test shape also does not follow the rules of Set B as there are three crescent shapes and four circular shapes present as opposed to the rule requiring four crescent shapes for every two circles.

Test Shape 4 – Set B

There are four circular shapes and two crescent shapes present, which therefore indicates that this test shape conforms to the rules of Set B. This shape does not follow the rules of Set A as there are six rectangular shapes to four circular shapes, whereas to follow the rule of this set it should comprise of four rectangular shapes and two circular shapes.

Test Shape 5 – Neither

The test shape contains six rectangular shapes and three circular shapes and therefore does not follow the rules of Set A, which must have four rectangular shapes to two circular shapes. The test shape also does not follow the pattern of Set B as there are four crescent shapes and three circular shapes present, when four crescent shapes to two circular shapes are required to follow the pattern of this set.

Question 10

Set A

There are various large symmetrical shapes which have been divided into five sections. Some of the divided sections are shaded in black while others are white.

There are three main rules for this set:

1. The outer shape should be symmetrical.

2. The shape should be divided into five parts.

3. The divided shape can be shaded in black or white.

Set B

There are various large symmetrical shapes present which have been divided into three sections. Some of the divided sections are shaded in black while others are white.

There are three main rules to this set which are:

1. The outer test shape should be symmetrical.

2. The shape should be divided into three parts.

3. The divided shape can be shaded in black or white.

Test Shape 1 – Set A

The outer test shape is symmetrical and is divided into five sections and therefore follows the rule of Set A. It does not follow the rules of Set B as it is not divided into three parts.

Test Shape 2 – Neither

The test shape is presented in 3D whereas all of the shapes in both sets are presented in 2D, therefore the test shape does not follow the rules of either set.

Test Shape 3 – Set A

The test shape is symmetrical and is divided into five sections, therefore following the rules of Set A. It is not related to Set B as the test shape is not divided into three parts.

Test Shape 4 – Set B

The test shape is symmetrical and is divided into three sections, therefore following the rules of Set B. It does not follow the rules of Set A as it is not divided into five parts.

Test Shape 5 – Neither

The test shape is not symmetrical and hence is not related to either set.

Question 11

Set A

In half of the boxes there are a group of four straight lined shapes including a five point star. In the second half of the set there are a group of four curved shapes with the fifth shape being the same five point star.

Set B

Set B uses similar shapes to Set A, however the difference is in their positioning and groupings. In each of the boxes there are either three straight lined shapes with one curved shape, or there are three curved shapes with one straight lined shape.

Test Shape 1 – Set B

The test shape belongs to Set B as there are three curved shapes (an oval, a circle and a crescent) with one straight lined shape (a five point star). The test shape cannot belong to Set A as it would need to contain four curved shapes instead of three.

Test Shape 2 – Neither

The test shape does not belong to either set as there is a four point star instead of a five point star.

Test Shape 3 – Set B

The test shape belongs to set b as there are 3 curved shapes (two ovals and one circle) with a straight lined shape (a five point star). The test shape cannot belong to set a as there need to be 4 curved shapes instead of 3.

Test Shape 4 – Neither

The test shape does not belong to Set A as the set contains slim rectangles, which is a characteristic of Set B. However, the test shape also cannot belong to Set B as there are no curved shapes present.

Test Shape 5 – Neither

As above, the test shape does not belong to either set, as there are only four straight lined shapes. This characteristic does not follow the rules of either set.

Question 12

Set A

This set comprises various large shapes in each box, including a circle, an arrow, a rectangle, a cross with arrows on its points, a boat shape and another conjoining arrow. There are medium and small sized circular shapes, star shapes and triangular shapes also present.

The rules for this set are as follows:

1. For every large shape there must be a corresponding triangle(s), which is either inside or outside the large shape.

2. Medium and small sized circles and stars are present.

Set B

This set has various large shapes present in each box, which consist of two rectangular, an oval shape, a curved rectangular shape, a lightning bolt, a box arrow and a stop sign.

There are medium and small sized star and triangular shapes present.

The rules for this set are as follows:

1. For every large shape there must be a corresponding rectangle(s) which is either inside or outside of the large shape.

2. Medium and small sized stars and triangles are present.

Test Shape 1 – Set A

The large test shape is divided into two. One section of this division is a triangle. The circular and star shapes are also present. Therefore this test shape follows the patterns of Set A. This test shape does not follow the rules of Set B, as there are no corresponding rectangular shapes within or outside the large shape. Together with this, Set B only has small stars present and no small circular shapes are used in this.

Test Shape 2 – Set B

The test shape is divided into five unequal parts. There are also stars within this test shape which are present within the pattern of Set B. This shape is not part of Set A as there are no corresponding triangular shapes together with circular shapes present.

Test Shape 3 – Set B

The test shape is divided into five parts, and one part of the division represents a rectangular shape. The other is a square which is quartered into triangles. There are also stars within this test shape, which are present only within Set B. This shape is not part of Set A, as there no circles present.

Test Shape 4 – Set A

The large test shape is divided into three triangles. The circular and star shapes are also present. This test shape does not follow the pattern of Set B as there are no corresponding rectangular shapes within or outside the large shape. Together with this, Set B only has small star shapes present – there are no small circular shapes present.

Test Shape 5 – Neither

The test shape initially looks like it belongs in Set A as the large shape, the circle, is divided into four parts with each part resembling a triangle. On closer inspection, we can see that the shape has a curved outline and therefore cannot be part of Set A. This test shape also cannot be related to Set B as there are no corresponding rectangles within or outside the large shape.

Question 13

Set A

Within this set there are straight lined symmetrical shapes which have been divided into three parts.

Set B

As above, the straight lined shapes are divided into three parts. However, the shapes are asymmetrical.

Test Shape 1 – Neither

The test shape cannot belong to either set as it is curved, therefore this does not follow the rules of either set.

Test Shape 2 – Set A

The test shape belongs to Set A as it is a straight lined symmetrical shape which is divided into three parts.

Test Shape 3 – Neither

The test shape does not belong to either set as it has a combination of both curved and straight lines.

Test Shape 4 – Set A

The test shape belongs to Set A as it is a straight lined symmetrical shape and is divided into three parts.

Test Shape 5 – Set A

As above, the symmetrical shape is made up of straight lines and is divided into three parts.

Decision Analysis answers and justifications

Question 1   **Answer B**

(A, ⊁), (A, 2), (6, 3)

The code combines the words *(Opposite, Happy), (Opposite, People), (Run, Building)*

Option A	Uses the word 'Building', but ignores the rules of the brackets of the opposite of 'Happy' and the opposite of 'People'.
Option B	**Is the correct answer. The opposite of 'Happy' is 'Sad', the opposite of 'People' is 'Person' or even 'One's self'. 'Run' is substituted for 'Scampered' and 'Building' is replaced by 'Home'.**
Option C	In this sentence 'Scampered' is used instead of 'Run', however the rules of the brackets are ignored as per option A.
Option D	This option uses all of the words and rules of the brackets apart from the word 'Run'.
Option E	Similar to options A and C, Option E uses the word 'Building', but ignores the rules of the brackets for the opposite of 'Happy' and 'People'.

Question 2   Answer E

(13, H, 1,) (15, H), 10

The code combines the words *(Ice, Merge, Sun), (Footprints, Merge), Water*

Option A	In this sentence the words 'Sun' and 'Water' are used in their original form. However this option ignores the words 'Merge', 'Ice' and 'Footprints' and introduces the word 'Reflected'.
Option B	Incorporates all of the words in the code except for the word 'Footprints'.
Option C	This option uses all of the words in the code. However, we need to use common sense when making the best logical decision. For example, is it really possible to find footprints on ice? Option E gives a much better interpretation as footprints are more likely to be present in the snow.
Option D	The words in the code are all used within this option but the sentence does not make logical sense.
Option E	**Is the correct answer. 'Merge' is substituted for the word 'Dissolved', 'Water' is substituted for 'Sea', and 'Ice' is substituted for 'Snow'. 'Sun' and 'Footprints' are kept in their original format.**

Question 3   Answer C

($\nearrow$, 2), (A, B), 6, 8

The code combines the words (*Daring, People*) (*Opposite, Decrease*), *Run, Danger*

Option A	Ignores the rules of the brackets, ignores the word 'Run' and introduces the word 'Risk'.
Option B	Ignores the rules of the brackets.
Option C	**Is the correct answer as all words in the code are used. The opposite of 'Decrease' is 'Increase', where 'Increase' has been replaced with the word 'More'. 'Daring' has been replaced with 'Courageous'.**
Option D	Uses all of the words in the code except for the word 'Run'.
Option E	Incorporates the words in the bracket but ignores the words 'People' and 'Run'.

Question 4   Answers A & C

(2, ♋), 3

The code combines the words (*People, Trusting*), *Building*

Option A	**Is one of the correct options. 'Building' is replaced by the word 'Church', 'People' is substituted for the word 'Public' and 'Trust' is kept in its original format.**

| Option B | Does not make as much logical sense as options A and C. |

Option C Is the second correct option. All of the words are present in their original format except for the word 'Building' which is replaced with 'Bank'.

Option D Ignores the word 'Building'.

Option E Uses all of the words in the code but introduces the word 'Sponsored'.

Question 5   Answer C

(2,●), (A, B,) 26

The code combines the words *(People, Intelligent), (Opposite, Decrease), Thought*

Option A Ignores the rule of the brackets detailing the opposite of the word 'Decrease'.

Option B Ignores the rule of the brackets detailing the opposite of the word 'Decrease'.

Option C Is the correct answer and makes the most logical sense. It uses all of the words and the rules within the code. 'People' and 'Intelligent' are present as 'Genius's', the opposite of 'Decrease' is 'Increase' and 'Thought' is replaced with the word 'Brain'.

Option D This sentence incorporates all of the words in the code but does not make logical sense.

| Option E | Again this option uses all of the words present in the code but does not make logical sense. |

Question 6   Answer D

(A, 19), I, 6, (20, 3), ☐

The code combines the words *(Opposite, He), Up, Run, (Structure, Building), Angry*

| Option A | Uses the word 'Down' instead of the word 'Up', so can be discounted. |

| Option B | Ignores the rules of the brackets for '(Opposite, He)', and uses the word 'Down' instead of the word 'Up'. |

| Option C | Ignores the rules of the brackets for '(Opposite, He)'. |

| **Option D** | **Is the correct interpretation of the code. This option uses all of the words and the rules of the brackets. 'Structure' is replaced by 'Stairs' of a building, and 'Angry' is replaced by the word 'Rage'.** |

| Option E | Uses the word 'Down' instead of 'Up', so can be discounted. |

Question 7   Answer C

(21, 2), (A, J), (A, 8), 2,

The code combines the words *(Security, People), (Opposite, Weak), (Opposite, Danger), People*

Option A	Ignores the words '(Security, People)'.
Option B	Ignores the words '(Security, People)' and 'Strong'.
Option C	**Is the correct answer. It uses all of the words in the code and makes logical sense. The words '(Security, People)' are replaced with 'Police' and 'Safeguards' and 'People' are replaced with 'Public'. The opposite of 'Weak' is 'Strong' and the opposite of 'Danger' is 'Safe'.**
Option D	Ignores the word 'Strong' and '(Security, People)'. This option also introduces the words 'Professional members'.
Option E	Introduces the words 'Structure' and ignores the codes for '(Security, People)', 'People' and 'Strong'.

Question 8   Answer B

5, 7, 11, 10

The code combines the words *Yesterday, Sand, Tomorrow, Water*

Option A	Uses all of the words in the code but the sentence has no logical meaning.
Option B	**Is the correct answer. The word 'Sand' is replaced by 'Dry' and 'Water' is replaced by 'Wet'. Remember the order of the words in the code do not necessarily have to appear in that specific order in the actual interpretation of the code.**

Option C	Ignores the word 'Tomorrow'.
Option D	Ignores the word 'Yesterday' and introduces the word 'Inside'.
Option E	Uses all of the words in the code but the sentence has no logical meaning.

Question 9   **Answers C & E**

4, (A, B), (A, D), 1, 10, 7

The code combines the words *City, (Opposite, Decrease), (Opposite, Cold), Sun, Water, Sand*

Option A	Introduces the word 'Shine' which is not present in the code and ignores the bracket '(Opposite, Cold)'.
Option B	Ignores the words 'Sand', 'Water' and introduces the words 'Sleep' and 'Shine' which are not contained within the code.
Option C	**Uses all of the words in the code. The word 'Beaches' replaces the code words 'Sun', 'Sea' and 'Sand'. 'Sunshine' is used instead of 'Warm'.**
Option D	Uses all of the words in the code but ignores the rule of the brackets for '(Opposite, Cold)'.
Option E	**Uses all of the words in the code. 'City' is replaced by 'Cairo', '(Opposite, Cold)' is replaced by the word 'Hot' and the word 'Water' is replaced by 'Sea'. The rest of the words used as presented in the code.**

Question 10   Answer C

22, 2, (A, ⌘, C), 8

The code combines the words *Natural, People, (Opposite, Unstable, Negative), Danger*

Option A	Ignores the rules of the brackets for '(Opposite, Unstable, Negative)'.
Option B	Introduces the word 'Liability'.
Option C	**Is the correct answer as it uses all of the words in the code. The code words 'Natural' and 'Danger' are replaced by 'Earthquake' which can be perceived as a natural disaster. The opposite of 'Unstable' is 'Calm', and 'Negative' is replaced with 'Never'.**
Option D	Ignores the rules of the brackets for '(Opposite, Unstable, Negative)'.
Option E	Ignores the rules of the brackets for '(Opposite, Unstable, Negative)'.

Question 11   Answer B

(2, A), (A, ◯, C), (◯), 2

The code combines the words *(People, Opposite), (Opposite, Extraverted, Negative), Extraverted, People*

Option A	Uses all of the words in the code but does not make logical sense.
Option B	**Is the correct answer as it uses all of the words in the code. The '(Opposite, People)' becomes 'I',**

	'(Opposite, Extraverted, Negative)' is replaced by 'Shy', 'Reserved' and 'Dislike'. 'Extraverted' is substituted for 'Sociable' and 'People' is kept in its original form.
Option C	Ignores the rules of the brackets for '(Opposite, Extraverted, Negative)' and ignores 'People'.
Option D	Ignores the rules of the brackets for '(Opposite, Extraverted, Negative)' and ignores 'People'.
Option E	Ignores the rules of the of the brackets for '(Opposite, Extraverted, Negative)'.

Question 12   Answer E

4, 10, 1, (22, 8)

The code combines the words *City, Water, Sun, (Natural, Danger)*

Option A	Introduces the word 'Countries' and also ignores the words 'City' and 'Sun'.
Option B	Ignores the code words 'City' and 'Sun' and also does not make logical sense.
Option C	Ignores the code word 'Sun'.
Option D	Uses all of the words contained in the code but does not make logical sense.

Option E	**Is the correct answer. Instead of 'City' the word 'London' is used. 'Water' is represented as 'Flood' which incorporates the meaning of 'Natural Danger' or a natural disaster. The 'Sun' is replaced with 'Dry'.**

Question 13   Answers B & C

2, (13, 3), D

The code combines the words *People, (Ice, Building), Cold*

Option A	Introduces the word 'Falls' and ignores the code word 'People'.
Option B	**Uses all of the code words but with various substitutes. 'People' is replaced with 'Residents', 'Building' is replaced with 'Homes', 'Ice' is replaced with 'Snow' and the word 'Cold' is indicated by 'Antarctic'.**
Option C	**Uses all of the code words. Instead of using the word 'People' the word 'Inuit people' is used who reside in 'Igloos' which replaces the meaning of '(Ice, Building)'.**
Option D	Introduces the word 'Freezer' and ignores '(Ice, Building)'.
Option E	Ignores the code words 'People' and 'Ice'.

Question 14   Answer E

(24, 1), 2, 9, ⋈

The code combines the words (*Colour, Sun*), *'People'*, *'Tonight'*, *'Happy'*

Option A	Introduces the word 'Face' and ignores the words 'Happy' and 'Tonight'.
Option B	Uses all of the words in the code but introduces the word 'Shone'.
Option C	Ignores the words 'People', 'Colour' and 'Happy'.
Option D	Ignores the words '(Colour, Sun)'.
Option E	**Is correct as it uses all of the words within the code. '(Colour, Sun)' are combined together as the sun can often change the colour of the sky. Therefore in the sentence, the sun has changed the sky 'Red'. 'Delight' is used instead of 'Happy' and finally 'Night' is used instead of 'Tonight'.**

Question 15   Answer B

(17, A), H, 4, (A, 1)

The code combines the words (*Light, Opposite*), *Merge, City, (Opposite, Sun)*

Option A	Ignores the word 'Merge'.
Option B	**Is correct as it uses all of the words provided within the code. Although the word 'Shyly' is added into the**

sentence, when we compare this option to the rest, this is the best choice, and gives the most logical explanation. 'Darkness' is used instead of '(Opposite, Light)' and 'Moon' is used instead of '(Opposite, Sun)'.

Option C	Ignores the rules of the brackets for '(Opposite, Sun)' and ignores 'Merge'.
Option D	Ignores the rules of the brackets for '(Opposite, Sun)' and ignores 'Merge'.
Option E	Ignores the rules of the brackets for '(Opposite, Sun)'.

Question 16   Answer D

20, ⌘, 3

The code combines the words *Structure, Unstable, Building*

Option A	Uses all of the words in the code but is not a logical interpretation.
Option B	Introduces the words 'Terrible state'.
Option C	Introduces the word 'Enormously'.
Option D	**Is the correct answer as all the code words are used. The words are replaced: 'Walls' is used to define 'Structure', 'Crumbling' is used to describe the house being 'Unstable', and finally 'House' is used instead of 'Building'.**
Option E	Ignores the word 'Building'.

Question 17   Answer E

22, 8, (G, 7)

The code combines the words *Natural, Danger, (Quickly, Sand)*

Option A	Uses all of the words in the code but also introduces the word 'Jungle'.
Option B	Introduces the word 'Jungle', and ignores the word 'Quickly'.
Option C	Introduces the words 'Jungle' and 'Run'.
Option D	Introduces the words 'Habitat' and 'Overflows'.
Option E	**Is the correct answer as it uses all of the words interpreted in different forms. '(Quickly, Sand)' are combined together to give 'Quicksand' and 'Natural' and 'Danger' are used together to give a natural disaster/ danger such as 'Quicksand' and is therefore the closest matching option.**

Question 18   Answer A

(A, J, 18), 2, ⚹

The code combines the words (*Opposite, Weak, Anatomy*), *People and Happy*.

Option A	**Is the correct answer as the word 'Healthy' is used to replace the '(Opposite, Weak)' and 'Body' is used instead of 'Anatomy'.**

Option B	Ignores the word 'Anatomy'.
Option C	Ignores the rules of the brackets for '(Opposite, Weak)'.
Option D	Introduces the word 'I' and ignores the code word 'People'.
Option E	Uses all of the words but does not make logical sense.

Question 19　　Answer C

(A, 2), (◆,⌘), 2, (C, ♋)

The code combines the words *(Opposite, People), (Shy, Unstable), People, (Negative, Trusting)*

Option A	Ignores the word 'Unstable'.
Option B	Ignores the words '(Opposite, People)' and 'Unstable'.
Option C	**Is the correct answer as it follows all of the rules in the brackets and uses all the code words. Some of the words are replaced: 'I' replaces '(Opposite, People)', 'Inhibited' and 'Unsteady' are used instead of '(Shy, Unstable)' and '(Negative, Trusting)' is replaced with 'Do not trust'.**
Option D	Ignores the words '(Negative, Trusting)' and 'Unstable'.
Option E	Introduces the word 'You' and ignores '(Opposite, People)' and 'Unstable'.

Question 20   Answer C

19, (A, 19), (C, ☺) ‚☐

The code combines the words *He, (Opposite, He), (Negative, Trusting), Angry*

Option A   Does not include the code words which describe the words 'He' and 'She' and introduces the code word for 'People'.

Option B   Does not include a code word which describes the word 'She', which is the '(Opposite, He)'.

Option C   Is the correct answer as the code provides the best interpretation of the sentence in the following way: "He' was hot-headed (Angry) as 'She' (Opposite, He) was not 'Trusting' (Negative, Trusting)".

Option D   Does not include code words which follow the rules of the brackets for '(Negative, Trusting)'.

Option E   As above, this code does not include words which follow the rules of the brackets for '(Negative, Trusting)'.

Question 21   Answer B

8, (22, 8, 25), 3, 20, (A, J)

The code combines the words *Danger, (Natural, Danger, Breeze), Building, Structure, (Opposite, Weak)*

Option A   Does not include code words to
                  describe the words 'Hurricane' or
                  'Buildings'.

**Option B   Is the correct answer as the code
                  words provide the best interpretation
                  of the sentence. 'Strong' replaces
                  '(Opposite, Weak)', 'Hurricane'
                  replaces '(Natural, Danger, Breeze)'.
                  The final part of the sentence,
                  "made the structure of the building
                  dangerous" is represented by the
                  code words 'Danger', 'Structure' and
                  'Building'.**

Option C   Does not a include code words for
                  'Hurricane'.

Option D   Does not include code words for
                  'Strong' and 'Hurricane', and a code
                  word for 'City' is introduced.

Option E   Does not include a code word for
                  'Hurricane' and uses the code word
                  'Weak' instead of 'Strong'.

Question 22   Answer C

(A, K), O, 2, (A, 2), O

The code combines the words *(Opposite, Hard),
Extraverted, People, (Opposite, People), Extraverted*

Option A   Uses all of the code words, however
                  does not follow the rules of the
                  brackets.

Option B   Ignores the code word for 'Easy'.

Option C	Is the correct answer as all of the code words used interpret the sentence correctly. "I (Opposite, People) find it easy (Opposite, Hard) to get on with self-assured (Extraverted) people (People) as I am gregarious (Extraverted) myself".
Option D	Does not include a code word for 'Easy'
Option E	Does not include code words for 'Easy or 'Extraverted'.

Question 23   Answer B

(A, 1), 2, 25

The code combines the following words *(Opposite, Sun), People, Breeze*

Option A	Does not make reference to 'Moon' and introduces the word 'I'.
Option B	Is the correct answer as the codes interpret the sentence in the following way: "'People (People) tend to float (Breeze) on the moon (Opposite, Sun)'.
Option C	Uses all of the code words, however there are no brackets present to convert the meaning of the word 'Sun' to 'Moon'.
Option D	Introduces the word 'Footprints'.
Option E	Does not include a code word for 'Breeze'.

Question 24   Answer D

(A, 2), (A, D), (C, L)

The code combines the words *(Opposite, People)*, *(Opposite, Cold)*, *(Negative, Desire)*

Option A	Uses all of the appropriate codes, however there are no brackets used to separate the meanings of each of the code words.
Option B	Introduces a code word for 'Colour'.
Option C	Does not include a code word for 'I' and uses the code for 'People' instead.
Option D	**Is the correct answer as the codes are translated in the following way: "I (Opposite, People), dislike (Negative, Desire) fire (Opposite, Cold) as it will burn (Opposite, Cold) me'.**
Option E	Does not include a code word for 'Dislike'.

Question 25   Answer: E

(C, L), 17, 18, (A, 2), 24

The code combines the words *(Negative, Desire)*, *Light*, *Anatomy*, *(Opposite, People)*, *Colour*

Option A	Does not include a code word for 'Dislike'.
Option B	Does not contain a code word for 'I'.
Option C	Uses all of the code words but does not follow the rules of the bracket to convert some of their meanings.

Option D   Introduces a code word for 'Sand'.

Option E   **Is the correct answer as the codes interpret the sentence in the following way: "I (Opposite, Person) dislike (Negative, Desire) my light (Light) coloured (Colour) eyes (Anatomy)".**

Question 26   **Answer A**

2, (C, L), 20, L, (A,⌘) ⌘, ↗

The code combines the words *People, (Negative, Desire), Structure, Desire, (Opposite, Unstable), Unstable, Daring*

Option A   **Is the correct answer as it interprets the sentence in the following way: "Audacious (Daring) people (People) prefer (Desire) change (Unstable) rather than structure (Structure) and stability (Opposite, Unstable)'.**

Option B   Uses all of the words in the code, however there are no brackets to convert the meanings of some of the code words.

Option C   Ignores the code word for 'People'.

Option D   Ignores the code word for 'People', and uses the singular 'I' instead.

Option E   Introduces the code word for 'Danger'.

Chapter 9

Closing Thoughts

The aim of this guide has been to provide you with an insight into the UKCAT and give you the opportunity to practice the various questions you will come up against. Our hope is that, by following the principles and steps contained in this guide, you will be able to confidently complete your UKCAT with excellent results.

If you feel that you still require further practice and would like to experience the UKCAT in an online format, you can subscribe to our online revision lessons at www.apply2.co.uk.

In addition to this guide, the Apply2Medicine and Apply2Dentistry websites (www.apply2medicine. co.uk and www.apply2dentistry.co.uk) contain lots of free resources, including details of 'hot topics' in the medical and dental world, to help you prepare for your application to Medical or Dental School and subsequent interview.

We strongly recommend that you do seek more information from the Medical or Dental Schools to which you are applying, and also from the official UKCAT websites, to ensure that you are fully prepared for your UKCAT.

From all at Apply2Medicine and Apply2Dentistry, we would like to wish you every success in securing your place at Medical or Dental School.

Good Luck!